Timeless

A Century of Iconic Looks

For my family.

An Hachette UK Company
www.hachette.co.uk

First published in Great Britain in 2017 by Mitchell Beazley, a division of
Octopus Publishing Group Ltd
Carmelite House
50 Victoria Embankment
London EC4Y 0DZ
www.octopusbooks.co.uk

ISBN 978 1 78472 370 5

Printed and bound in China

10 9 8 7 6 5 4 3

Commissioning Editor Joe Cottington
Art Director Yasia Williams-Leedham
Make-up Louise Young
Hair Loulia Sheppard
Photography Denisa Ilie
Assistant Madeleine White
Illustrations Cate Wicks
Senior Editor Alex Stetter
Copy Editor Zia Mattocks
Senior Production Controller Allison Gonsalves

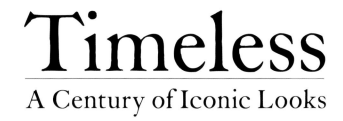

Timeless

A Century of Iconic Looks

Recreate the
classic make-up
and hair styles from
100 years of beauty

LOUISE YOUNG
WITH LOULIA SHEPPARD

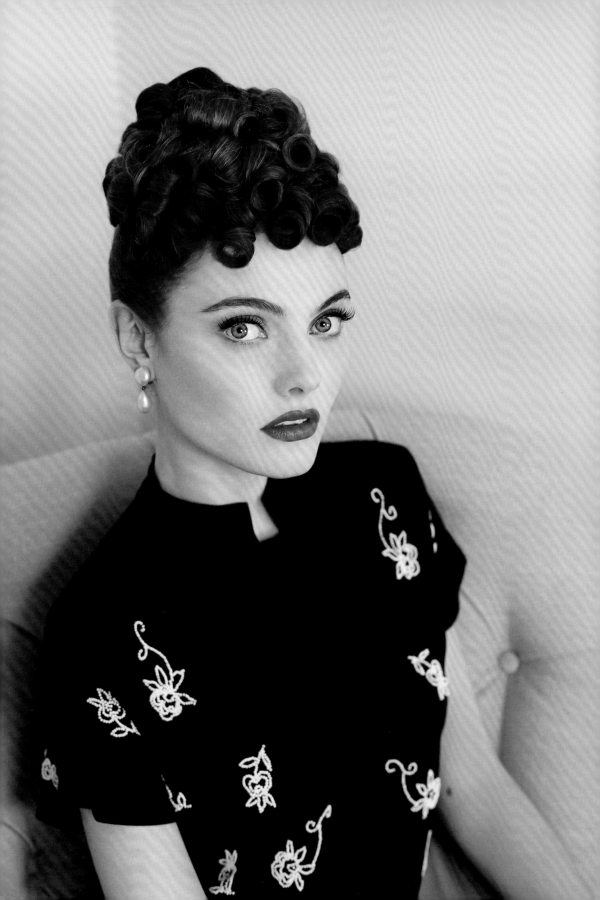

Contents

Introduction   6

The Early Years   10

The 1930s   44

The 1940s   66

The 1950s   128

The 1960s   162

The 1970s   202

The 1980s and Beyond   226

Index   250

Acknowledgements   255

About the Authors   256

Opposite: An iconic 1940s look (see page 90)

Introduction

FOR AS LONG AS I CAN REMEMBER, I HAVE BEEN PASSIONATE ABOUT MAKE-UP. I AM FORTUNATE TO HAVE HAD A CAREER AS A MAKE-UP ARTIST FOR NEARLY 40 YEARS NOW, DOING SOMETHING I LOVE. I HAVE WORKED IN ALL AREAS OF THE BUSINESS, FROM FILM AND TELEVISION TO FASHION, THEATRE AND SPECIAL EFFECTS.

As a child I was fascinated by old Hollywood, and I 'made up' the glamorous stars in the film annuals and magazines I collected by drawing on extra eyelashes and fuller lips with crayons. I instinctively wanted to make up people's faces, but was not yet aware of the career options available. I could often be found reading biographies of the stars from the silent era and beyond, and spent many afternoons watching Fred Astaire and Ginger Rogers dancing across the screen, laughing at the Marx Brothers and admiring the beauty of Marilyn Monroe and Audrey Hepburn. There were posters of Steve McQueen and Paul Newman on my bedroom wall, and I dreamt of getting to meet them one day.

By the time I was 13 I had a wide-reaching knowledge of the films and stars of Hollywood's golden years. Along with my love of music and fashion, this background knowledge has been invaluable in my work as both a make-up artist and a teacher. I have lectured in media make-up for more than 25 years and have taught many successful make-up artists working today.

Owing to the overwhelming amount of conflicting information and images available on the Internet and in books and magazines, it can be very easy for people to become confused about what is historically accurate and what is someone else's interpretation of a look from the past.

I have found that in many cases the looks of entire decades have been distorted. This is why I have long wanted to create a resource for make-up and hair enthusiasts, students and professionals alike, that was reliable and thoroughly researched – something that was true to the times it depicted.

The catalyst that actually made this book happen was working on a film three years ago with Loulia Sheppard, a hairstylist with 40 years' experience, who can create styles from any era. Lou and I were chatting about the fact that, as with any subject, it is important to learn from the past in order to understand the present – hence why watching old films, learning about the politics of the time and getting to know your references is so invaluable when recreating vintage styles. I mentioned that I was writing a book and asked Lou to do the hair. I knew I had found the right person for this project, as Lou is widely regarded as one of the best period hairstylists in the business – though she is very modest and won't like me saying this! She has worked with some of the biggest stars in the industry and created some of the most spectacular hairstyles on film. She teaches masterclasses for industry professionals, and her knowledge and skills are highly sought after.

Over the past two years, in between working on films, Lou and I worked on all the shoots for this book, carefully choosing the models to try and capture the correct feel of each era. Every look is accompanied by a reference picture showing a similar look from the decade in question. To add to the accuracy, the clothes the models are wearing are authentic vintage garments from that time.

In the step-by-step instructions for the make-up and the hair, Lou and I have tried to make recreating the looks as simple as possible.

Opposite: A simple 1940s look (see page 124)

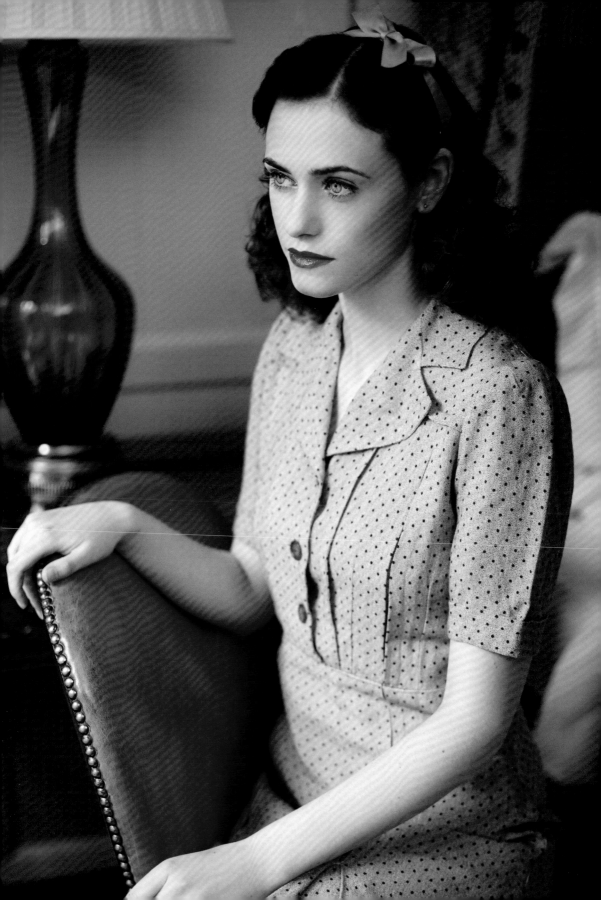

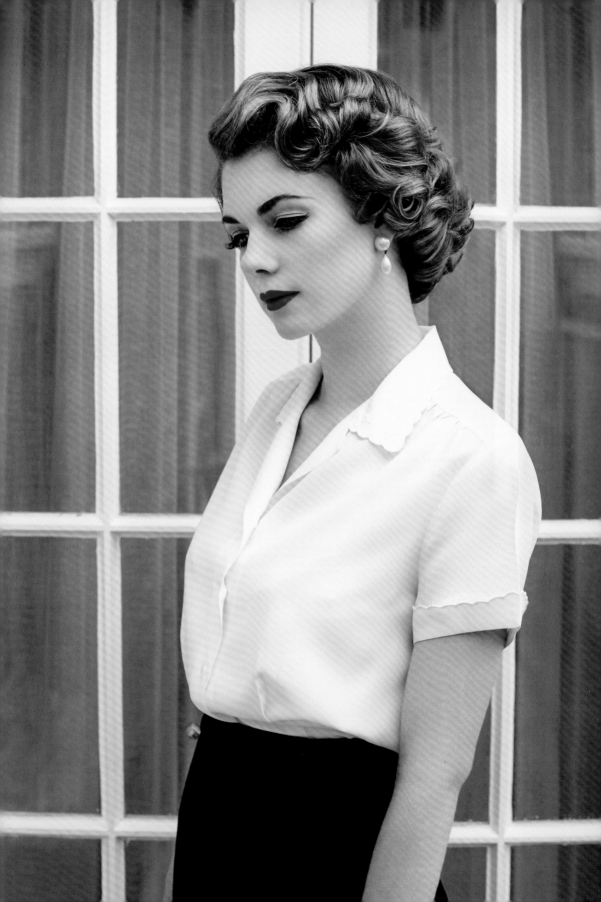

In many cases we have included variations for both hair and make-up – sometimes a small change can create a completely different look. When teaching make-up, I make sure my students understand light and shade, and how this can alter the face, enlarging or minimizing an area, lifting an eye or drooping it. Once you understand these basic techniques, you can do any look. In the same way, Lou emphasizes that if you take the time to get the hair set right in the first place, the style will be much easier to achieve. We also included many of the tips and tricks we have learnt from experience over the years that will transform a look from ordinary to amazing.

I hope this book will appeal to people on a variety of levels. It can serve as a reference for those wanting to accurately recreate a look from the past, whether they are students or professionals, but it will be just as useful to the many women who love vintage clothes and want to complete the look with the right hair and make-up – and this book shows you how to do that. I believe the book will also appeal to anyone who just wants to add a touch of vintage inspiration – a little Hollywood glamour, perhaps – to their look, without going the whole way. The looks we have chosen can be adapted to work in a modern setting as well.

I also hope this book will be useful to anyone with an interest in understanding how we got where we are today in terms of make-up and hair fashions. The forever-evolving timeline of make-up, hair and fashion is something that everyone can relate to, as this is how we represent ourselves to the outside world, and how we tell our story every morning as we get ready for the day.

So often, the social history of an era was part and parcel of the development of trends in make-up and hair.

Throughout the book I have referenced not just the people who influenced the looks and styles of the day, but also the products and social factors that were important in their evolution. Each chapter features a selection of make-up and hair products from the era, some of which come from our personal collections and some from the London Cosmetics Museum, to which we are very grateful for allowing us to photograph them. These items offer a fascinating insight into the time, from the small, camera-shaped compacts from the 1930s, which held all the cosmetics a woman might want to carry in her tiny, elegant purse on a night out, to the patriotic packaging introduced to boost morale during the Second World War. Advertisements also offer a great insight into what kinds of looks were deemed to be acceptable or considered to be desirable. One only has to look at some of the early cosmetics advertisements to see the social changes that have taken place, from the attitudes towards 'respectable' women wearing make-up at all to the development of safer ingredients.

I hope this information will be useful for anyone wanting to do further research, as it is always best to go back to a source from the time, rather than just searching the web for '1940s make-up', for instance. Instead, look up a specific actress or actor of the period – I have named many of my favourites in this book – and that will provide you with starting points for further research.

Be aware that the 'Hollywood' version of a woman's look was generally more glamorous than the 'real thing'.

To get the look of an average woman in wartime, for instance, search for pictures of women taken at the time, perhaps working in factories or out in the streets. The more glamorous looks in this book can easily be toned down to create a look that a normal girl would wear: leave off the false lashes, just put a stain on the lips and do a simpler version of the hair.

I do hope you enjoy the book and recreating the looks we have selected. It has been a pleasure to research, write about and bring alive some of our favourite historical looks, and it would not have been possible without the amazing team we had.

Opposite: A classic 1950s look (see page 140)

The Early Years

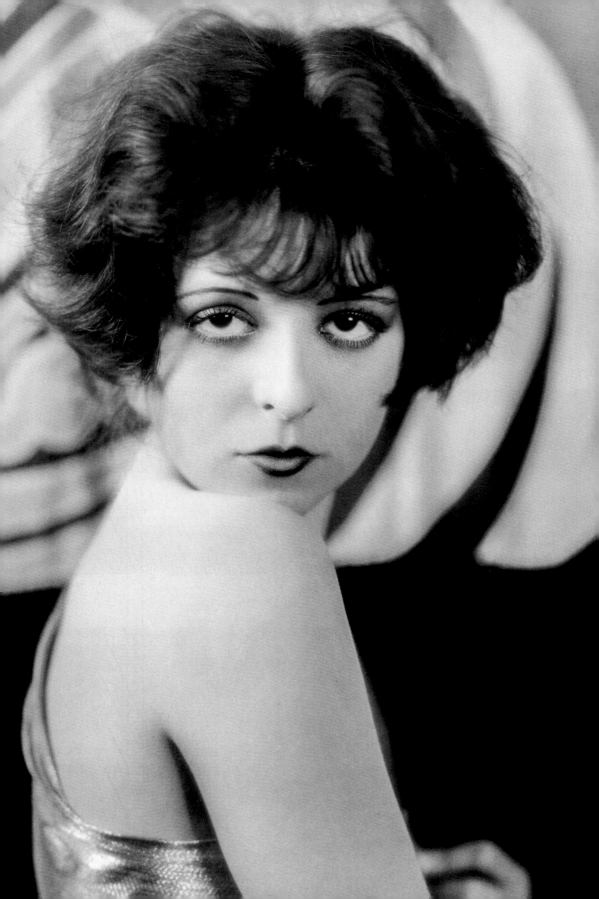

The Early Years

BY THE 1920S, WOMEN HAD BEEN FREED FROM THE RESTRICTIVE CLOTHING AND SOCIAL LIMITATIONS OF THE EARLY 20TH CENTURY, AND THIS DEVELOPMENT WAS REFLECTED IN THE HAIR AND MAKE-UP STYLES OF THE ERA.

The custom that respectable women did not wear make-up lasted into the early 20th century. But by the 1920s make-up was much more popular, though still viewed with suspicion by some.

MAKE-UP

During the first decade of the 20th century the use of powder and a little rouge (blusher) was largely accepted, as long as the resulting look was natural and the make-up was undetectable in daylight. Women paid a great deal of attention to skincare, using face creams, masks and skin whiteners that promised to deliver the desired youthful glow. As ingredients were unregulated, there were many resulting cases of damage to the skin. The quest for the perfect complexion continued after 1910, and by the middle of the decade rouge was available in paste, liquid and cake form.

As the Women's Suffrage Movement grew, some women wore lip rouge to make a political statement. The First World War (1914–18) brought dramatic changes in fashion, while new attitudes to the use of cosmetics also emerged.

Then came the Roaring Twenties, a term that evokes the fast and furious lifestyle of a certain section of society: the Flappers, the fashionable, fun-loving young women who rejected the conventions of the previous generation. Their distinctive look is the one most people associate with the decade: the bobbed hair, pale skin, dark eyes and Cupid's bow mouth of silent era film stars such as Louise Brooks, Clara Bow and Mae Murray. After the almost secretive approach to wearing make-up that prevailed at the start of the century, these bold style icons of the 1920s represented change and emancipation for women.

Max Factor brought make-up off the silver screen and on to women's faces in a form that was easier to apply and wear than the heavy formulas developed for use under the bright lights of a film set. In the 1920s he created a range of cosmetics called Society Makeup, so named in order to confer on the products an air of respectability.

Arch rivals Helena Rubinstein and Elizabeth Arden were already successful businesswomen by the 1920s, owning salons across the USA. They soon both moved into producing products and continued to be innovative leaders in the make-up industry throughout their lives.

HAIR

At the beginning of the 20th century, hairstyles were soft and large, often padded out with hair collected from the hairbrush. These styles, which supported the huge hats that were fashionable at the time, were given even more volume with the use of false pieces known as transformations.

By 1918 women had started to trim the sides of their hair and dress the back in a chignon. In the 1920s many took the plunge and cut their hair short. From straight to wavy bobs, these sharp, audacious styles came to signify the new-found freedom of the 1920s woman. Androgynous fashions were reflected in styles such as the Eton crop, a short boyish cut worn slicked down by, for example, the American-born French singer and dancer Josephine Baker.

Opposite: Clara Bow, 1926

Achieving a beautiful complexion was considered to be of the utmost importance in the early years of the 20th century. As the use of make-up began to be socially acceptable, a burgeoning cosmetics industry soon appeared. Max Factor had created a flexible greasepaint for use in film and he began selling eyeshadow and brow pencils to the general public as early as 1916. His innovative products made him a leading name in cosmetics.

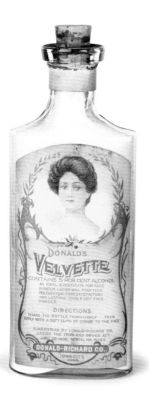

Eyelash beading ▲

A theatre technique adopted by film stars and some brave members of the public, beading involved melting a cosmetic wax and applying it to the lashes, leaving a small bead at the end of the clumped-together lashes.

Maybelline mascara ▼

Tom Lyle Williams is credited with inventing mascara in 1915. The company was named after his sister Mabel, who coated her lashes with Vaseline and cork ash. Originally 'Lash-Brow-Ine', it was one of the first commercial eye cosmetics.

Donald's Velvette ▲

Various preparations were available in the early 20th century to satisfy women's quest for perfect skin, from liquid powder, such as Donald's Velvette, to face whiteners, cold creams and skin tonics.

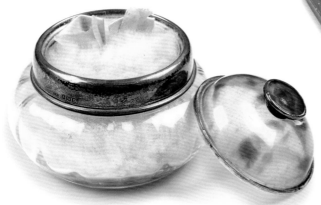

◀ **Face powder**

Often applied with a swansdown puff, face powder was initially available in White, Pink and Rachel, with other colours subsequently being introduced. It was often kept in ornate containers, which graced the dressing tables of Edwardian women.

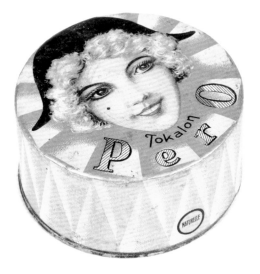

Ojos Negros powder ▲

This Argentinian face powder dates from 1927. The elegant Art Deco packaging features an illustration of a woman with the dark-rimmed eyes and small, deep red mouth that exemplify the 1920s look.

Tokalon loose powder ▲

This powder came in ten colours including Blanche (white), Naturelle (pink), Rachel (cream) and Brun Soleil (tan). In the late 1920s powders were starting to be available in colours to accommodate the newly fashionable sun-tanned skin.

Marcel irons ▲

Invented by Marcel Grateau in the early 1870s, the Marcel technique gained popularity during the late 19th century and was widely used until the late 1920s.

Gladys Cooper face powder ▲

Dame Gladys Cooper was a successful stage and screen actress of the early 20th century. Known as a great beauty, she had her own range of beauty preparations, such as this powder from the mid-1920s.

French shingling clipper ▶

The shingle haircut involved the hair at the nape of the neck being trimmed into a V-shape, close to the scalp, with the sides waved or curled. Also called the 'boyish bob', it caused a sensation when it first appeared in the early 1920s.

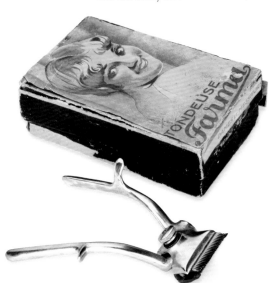

At the start of the 20th century, many products and home-made preparations promised the desired porcelain complexion, with some sold as virtual cure-alls for any beauty problem. Many advertisements included the words 'non poisonous' – an indication of the problems that arose due to the lack of testing and regulation. As the use of make-up became more widespread, the dramatic *femme fatale* look of actresses Theda Bara and Musidora from around 1915 heralded the arrival of the modern emancipated woman of the 1920s.

LIPSTICK

Tangee lipstick was hugely popular: it looked orange (hence the name), but on the lips it appeared anything from rose to a deep blush. The company's advertising claimed that every woman could wear Tangee lipstick because it changed colour to suit each individual complexion. Also popular lipstick colours were dark red, plum red, raspberry and carmine. In 1928, Max Factor created the forerunner of lipgloss, calling his pioneering product Lip Pomade.

EYESHADOW

Max Factor advertised eyeshadow in blue, brown and grey. Black, navy and dark green were also popular shades. For daytime, a dab of Vaseline (pictured top row, left) was often all that was worn on the lids. Pencils were also available to smudge around the eyes.

BLUSHER

Rouge for the cheeks was available as a paste or in powder form. Colours were advertised with names such as Egyptian Poppy, Rosebud and Vermilion, while Max Factor offered Carmine, Blondeen, Raspberry, Natural and Day rouge, among other shades. Red, rose and plum were popular colours.

In the 1920s, many women copied the dark eyes and lips of silent film stars.

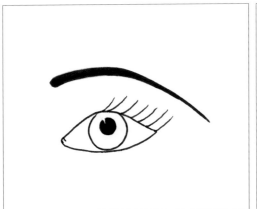

Brows

In the 1920s, the fuller, more natural eyebrows of the early 1900s gave way to some of the most extreme looks of the 20th century, as women copied the brows of their favourite film stars. Little or no attempt seems to have been made to create a natural brow. Eyebrows were plucked or shaved, and then new browlines were drawn on in their place. The popular brows of the day were pencil-thin and extended down to the temples, lending a mournful appearance to the eyes. While many brows were arched, some were straighter, for example those worn by Louise Brooks and Theda Bara.

Lips

Small lips with a prominent Cupid's bow were the fashion. Dark lip colours exaggerated this trend, making the lips appear smaller. Lip stencils were available to achieve this neat shape, but many women just took their preferred dark lip colour and applied it on the inner part of the lips only, avoiding taking it to the outer edge, thus making the lips appear smaller.

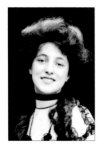

Created by American graphic artist Charles Dana Gibson in 1890, the Gibson Girl came to represent the ideal of American beauty of the time. With her hair piled high on top of her head in a soft pompadour style, her look became much imitated by models and actresses, including Camille Clifford and Evelyn Nesbit. Our reference picture shows Nesbit, who modelled for Gibson's drawing of 1905, *Woman: The Eternal Question*. Here, we show you a simple version of a typical Gibson Girl style. These hairstyles were also popular in Edwardian Britain and the rest of Europe, with Parisian women leading the way.

THE

EARLY

YEARS

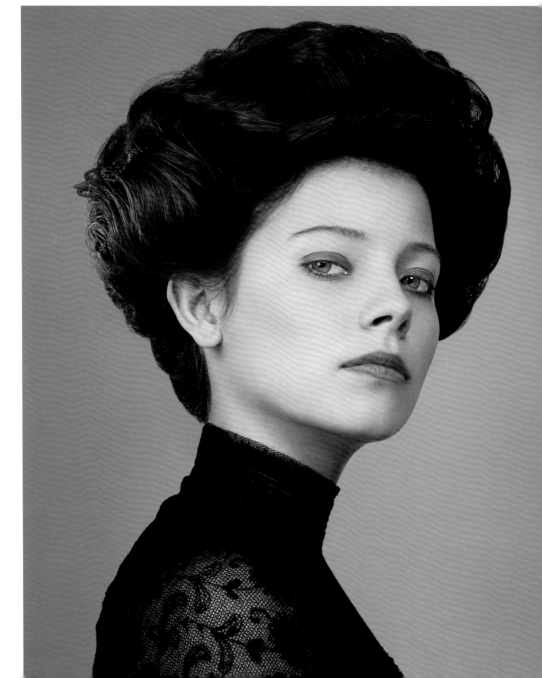

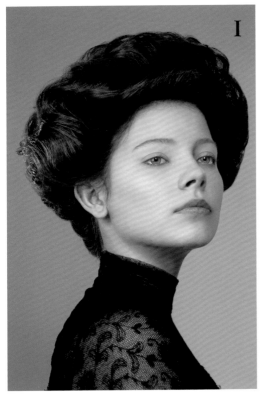

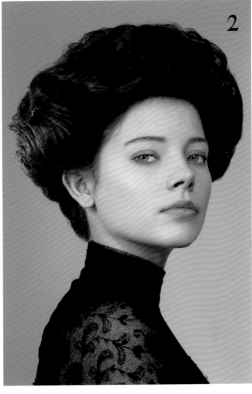

Step 1

Foundation: Apply a liquid or cream foundation using a foundation brush. Choose a colour that exactly matches the skin; mix two shades together if necessary to achieve a perfect match. I always stop at the jawline when applying foundation – I never take it under the jaw. If you are using the correct colour, there will be no visible line. The foundation should look like skin, not make-up.

Concealer: Apply concealer to any blemishes on the face with a small brush, choosing a shade that matches the skin colour. Use a lighter shade for under-eye shadows and apply the product only to the dark areas. Never apply concealer to the lighter, puffy areas as you will make them look more prominent.

Powder: Apply loose transparent powder all over the face using a puff and then remove the excess using a large, fluffy powder brush. Make sure the powder is completely colourless, otherwise you will be adding another layer of colour to the foundation.

Step 2

Eyeshadow: While the emphasis was on creating a beautiful complexion, some images from the time show the use of shading of the eyes and brows. Very lightly shade on the eye with a matte shadow in a neutral colour.

Brows: If necessary fill the brows to a natural shape with matte shadow using an angled brush.

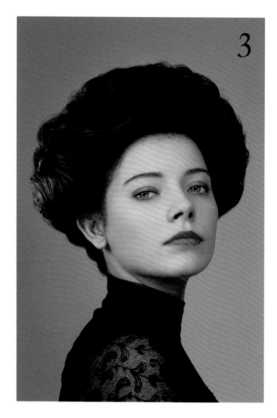

3

Step 3

Blusher: Using a soft blusher brush, apply powder blusher in a soft rose pink to the centre of the cheeks and blend very well.

In the early years of the 20th century, ladies liked their make-up to be completely undetectable in daylight. At the time, a coloured loose powder would have been applied on top of a face cream – the cream 'gripped' the powder, thus creating a foundation. Rouge was then applied to the cheeks. If it appeared too bright, another layer of powder would be applied to tone it down, until the ideal pink-and-white complexion had been achieved.

Lipstick: To give a neutral stain to the lips, apply lipstick in a shade matching the natural lip colour and then wipe it off to leave the merest hint of colour.

In the early 1900s, hair was generally dressed off the face and featured large pompadours, either smooth or waved.

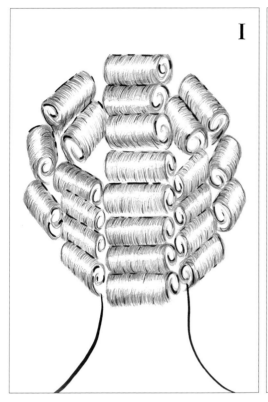

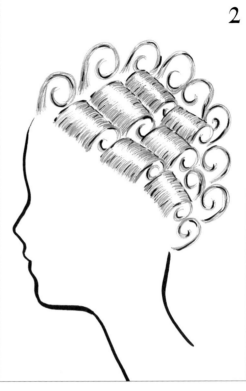

Step 1

For best results, the hair should not be freshly washed and conditioned, but 'day-old hair' – that is, washed the day before. If the hair is fine, use a mousse to give it some texture.

Using a tail comb, section the hair evenly around the head. Spray setting lotion on each section before setting the hair with heated rollers, as shown above. Leave to cool.

The size of the roller will determine the amount of wave: the larger the roller, the smoother the style, with less of a wave. For this look, Lou used medium-sized rollers and sectioned the hair as shown above, and set it in the direction she wanted to comb out the style.

Step 2

Take the rollers out when they are completely cool and lightly brush the hair through.

To style, put some padding on the crown of the head. Lou used crepe hair, which is soft and light to wear. You can also use shop-bought hair padding, such as doughnut bun rings. These are useful if you want to complete the look with a hat, as you can pin into this stiffer padding to secure the hat.

The aim is to brush the hair carefully in towards the crown, being careful not to dislodge the padding. You can do this in sections if you can't cope with all the hair at once. Start with the back, then the sides and lastly the front, backcombing each section to give extra bulk and lift.

As you push the hair up towards the crown, relax the tension on the hair slightly: you will see the waves form automatically – pin these into place.

Finish with a fine mist of hair spray.

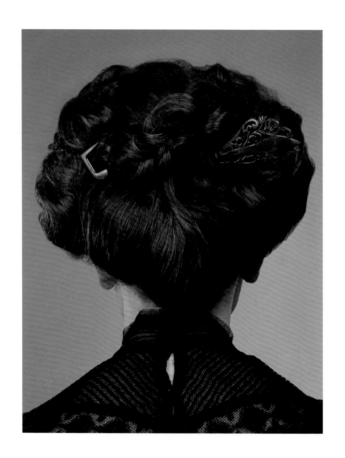

Often kept in place with ornate hair
combs, the hairstyles of this era
would also be adorned with feathers
and bows. Young girls wore their
hair down, tied with a ribbon.

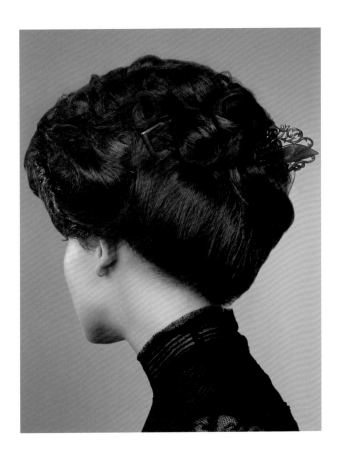

For a more casual, modern version
of the Gibson Girl style, pull out
some tendrils to frame the face
– this would work beautifully as
a bridal look today.

The ideal beauty of the Edwardian era had a clear complexion of pale ivory and pink, often achieved by layering powder, rouge and then more powder over a base of face cream.

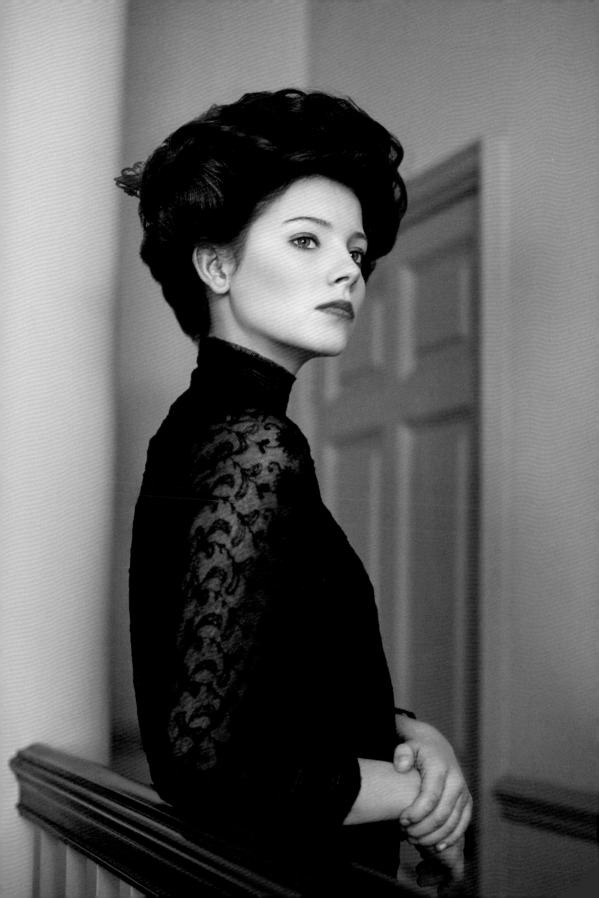

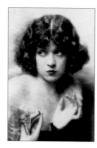

The original vamp, Theda Bara, was given her stage name and an exotic backstory by the Fox Film Corporation, one of the big film studios of the time. In 1915, the silent star epitomised the look of the sultry, brooding 'vampire woman'. By the time the 1920s arrived women had refined the vamp look somewhat, but the dark-rimmed eyes standing out against rouged, pale porcelain skin, with a small, dark mouth, still came to sum up the face of the decade. Our reference image shows Canadian-born screen actress Marie Prevost, a popular leading lady of the 1920s.

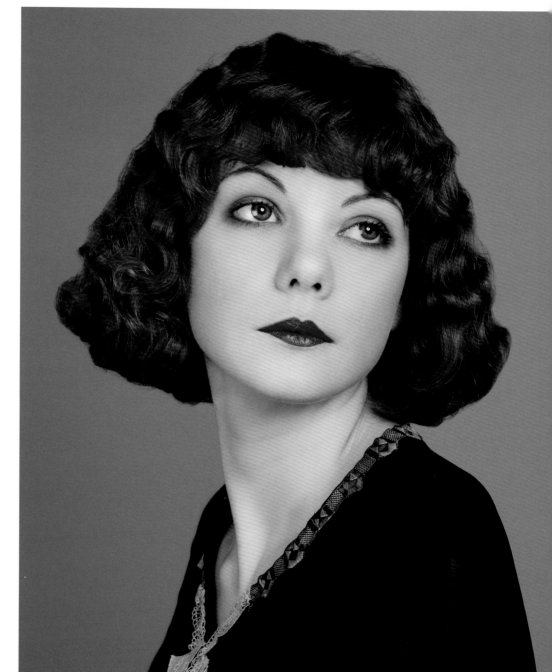

THE

EARLY

YEARS

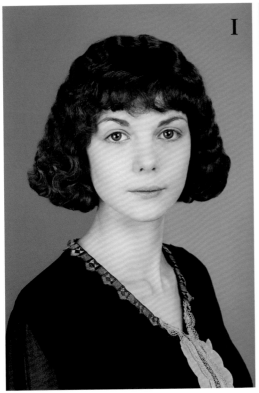

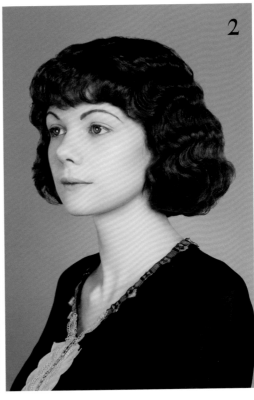

Step 1

Foundation: Apply foundation, followed by concealer and powder, as described in step 1 on page 19.

Step 2

Brows: To give our model's brows the thin 1920s shape, I started by blocking out the areas I wanted to disguise using a hard household soap. To do this, wet a spoolie or a clean disposable mascara brush and lather the soap to a paste. Apply this to the hairs on the underside of the brow first and then on the top, making sure they are coated in soap. Press the brow flat to the skin with your finger and allow it to dry (this doesn't take long). Cover the area you are blocking with camouflage cream mixed to the same colour as the skin. Powder the area well with colourless loose powder. Using a cake liner (as I have here) or a pencil, draw in the thin brows and extend them down onto the temples. You can find various images showing the different eyebrow shapes of the era, including brows coming right down onto the temples, very thin arches, and brows drawn on very low, just above the eyes.

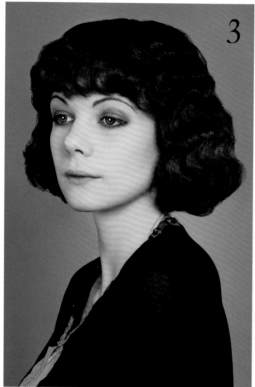

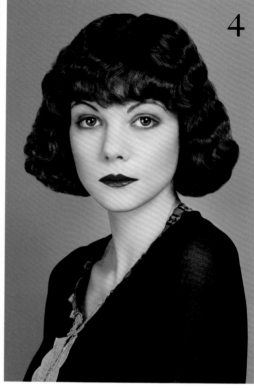

Step 3

Eyeshadow: Apply dark blue-grey shadow over the eyelid, keeping the half-moon shape and not winging the shadow up. Then take it under the eye, just below the roots of the lashes. This will create the typical doleful look that was popular. Soften the edges of the shadow with a blending brush.

Mascara: Apply black mascara to top and bottom lashes.

Step 4

Blusher: Apply blusher in a deep carmine-red shade to the apples of the cheeks, and blend it out.

Lipstick: Apply lip colour in dark red to create a small 1920s-style mouth with a pronounced Cupid's bow. To create the shape, first make the mouth look smaller by using a little powder foundation at the sides of the mouth to block out the areas you want to hide. Draw in the outline using a lip pencil in the same shade as the lipstick, making sure the shape is symmetrical, then fill it in and apply lipstick to the inner shape.

Although at the time lip stencils were available so women could achieve the perfect Cupid's bow, in reality this can look quite strange if you have a large, full mouth. The method of blocking out the outer edges of the mouth with foundation creates a more natural effect.

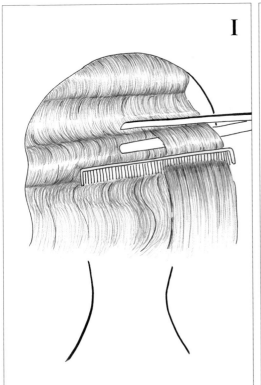

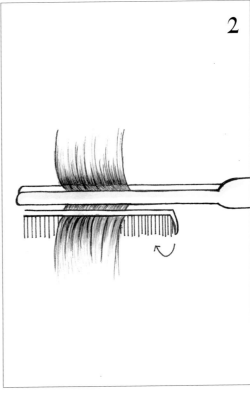

This hairstyle is achieved with small Marcel irons.

Step 1

With a comb in one hand and the iron held horizontally in the other, place the iron into a section of the hair. The cup of the iron should be on the underneath of your section and the barrel on the top. Place comb in the hair below the iron and direct the hair either left or right with the comb depending on which way you want the first wave to go. To make the wave, roll the iron up half a turn, hold a couple of seconds and roll down and remove iron.

Step 2

To set the direction of the next wave, place the iron in the section of hair directly under the crest of the wave, place the comb under the iron and push the comb to the opposite direction of the crest above using a small sweeping motion.

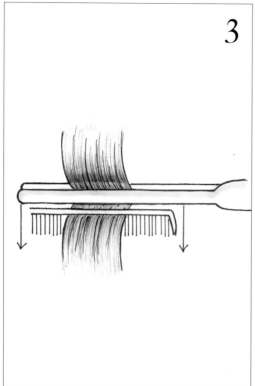

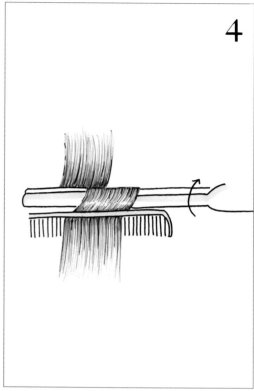

Step 3

Slide both the iron and the comb a little way down the hair in one smooth motion.

In the 1920s, the waves were quite small, so hardly any downwards movement is needed, but for larger, 1930s-style waves, slide the iron down about 1.5–2cm (½–¾ in).

Step 4

Roll the Marcel iron upwards a couple of turns then roll down and remove the iron.

This completes a wave. Lou does this as part of a continuous movement – this take a little practice!

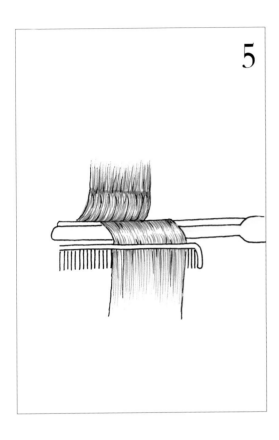

5

Step 5

To carry on waving the hair, reposition the iron below the crest of the next wave and repeat the previous steps, alternating the direction in which you push the comb on every wave. Continue the process all the way down each section of hair. Make sure not to drag the hair down while doing the waves: keep the tension relaxed, so you can always see the wave above while doing the next one.

The 1930s saw finger waves come into fashion, but Marcel waves were still worn by some women after the 1920s.

The Marcel wave was popular
from the late 19th century until
the late 1920s, propelling its
inventor, Marcel Grateau,
to fame and fortune.

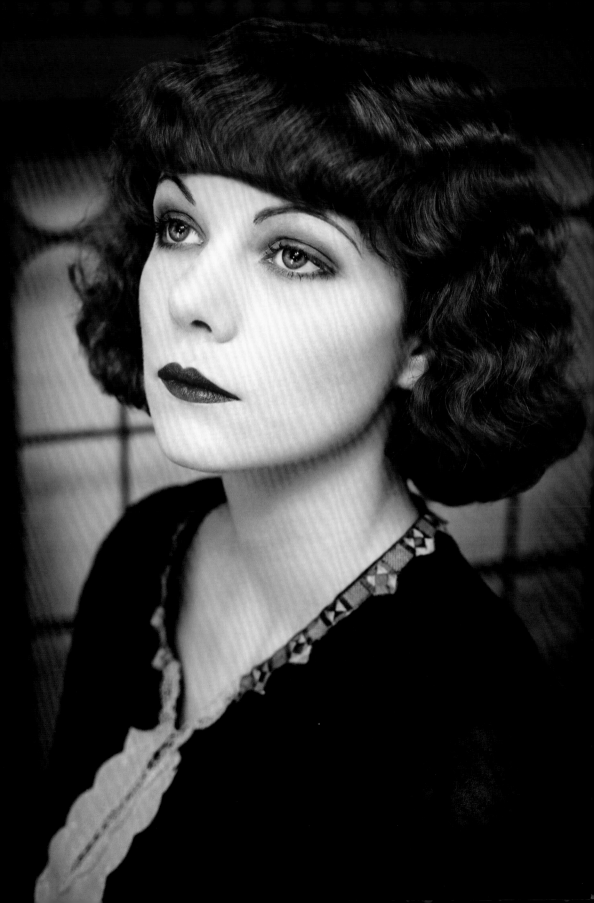

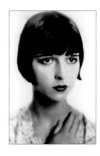

One of the first bobbed hairstyles appeared around 1915, as worn by ballroom dancer Irene Castle. Dubbed the Castle bob, the style wasn't widely adopted until the 1920s, when many fashionable women took the plunge and followed suit – no doubt encouraged by stars such as Louise Brooks (pictured) with her very short, straight bob and Clara Bow with her curly bob. Louise Brooks starred in a number of Hollywood films in the 1920s, and her stylish look with her ultra-short bob remains a lasting image of the Flapper era.

THE

EARLY

YEARS

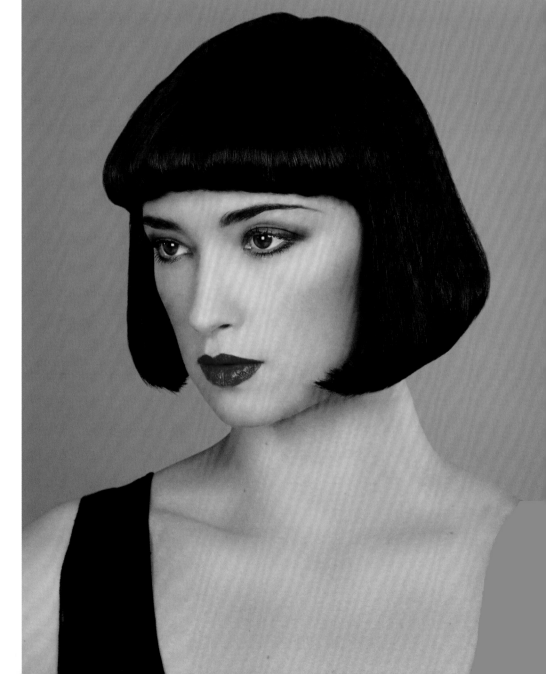

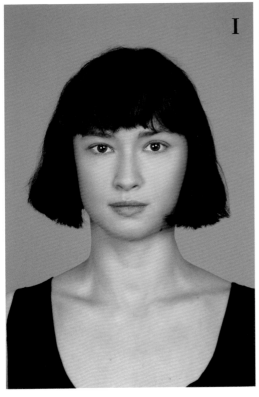

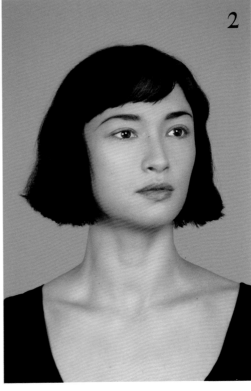

Step 1

Foundation: Apply a liquid or cream foundation using a foundation brush. Choose a colour that exactly matches the skin; mix two shades together if necessary to achieve a perfect match. I always stop at the jawline when applying foundation – I never take it under the jaw. If you are using the correct colour, there will be no visible line. The foundation should look like skin, not make-up.

Concealer: Apply concealer with a small brush. Use a lighter shade for under-eye shadows and apply the product only to the dark areas. Never apply concealer to the lighter, puffy areas as you will make them look more prominent. Apply concealer to any blemishes on the face, choosing a shade that matches the skin colour.

Powder: Apply loose transparent powder all over the face using a puff and then remove the excess using a powder brush. Make sure the powder is completely colourless, otherwise you will be adding another layer of colour to the foundation.

Step 2

Brows: There were a number of different brow shapes that were popular in the era. These, like Louise Brooks's, are a straighter style, thicker at the beginning and tapering to the outer corners. Use a cake liner to define and extend the brows out to the temples.

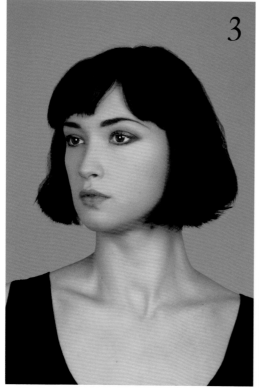

3

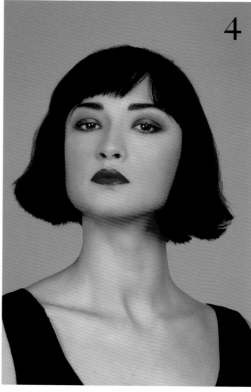

4

Step 3

Eyeshadow: Apply a dark grey cream shadow over the eyelids and underneath the bottom lashes, taking it out slightly beyond the outer corners. Lightly powder this with colourless loose powder to set the cream shadow.

Mascara: Apply mascara to the top and bottom lashes.

Step 4

Blusher: Apply a little powder blusher in a dark rose colour to the apples of the cheeks and blend it softly outwards.

Lipstick: Apply a deep red lipstick to complete the look.

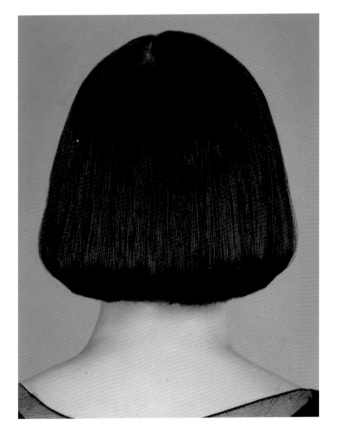

Hair

Smooth the hair into a sharp,
straight bob using a small
straightening iron. When you reach
the bottom of each strand, curve
the ends under all round.

Finish with a fine mist of hair spray.

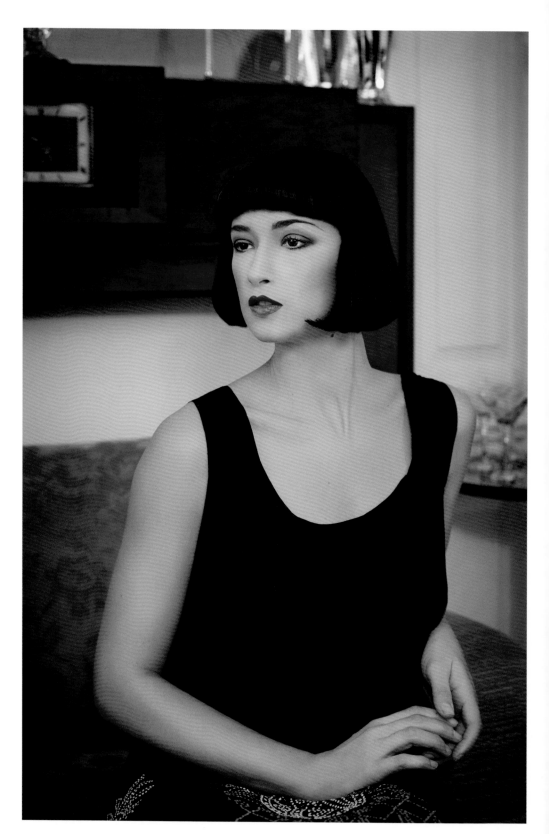

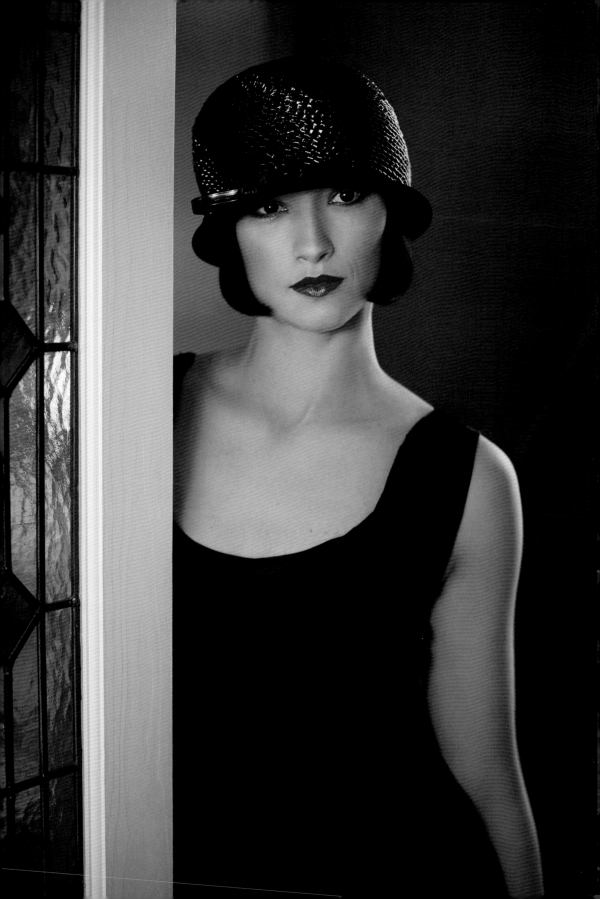

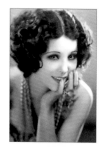

There was a strong fascination with ancient Egyptian culture in the 1920s, which was reflected in the clothes, jewellery and architecture of the decade. Women were already darkening their eyes and used kohl and liners to achieve an exotic, smouldering look, and the discovery in 1922 of Tutankhamun's tomb only fuelled this obsession and helped to heighten the practice. Our reference for this look is Raquel Torres, who appeared in a number of Hollywood films in the late 1920s and early 1930s.

THE

EARLY

YEARS

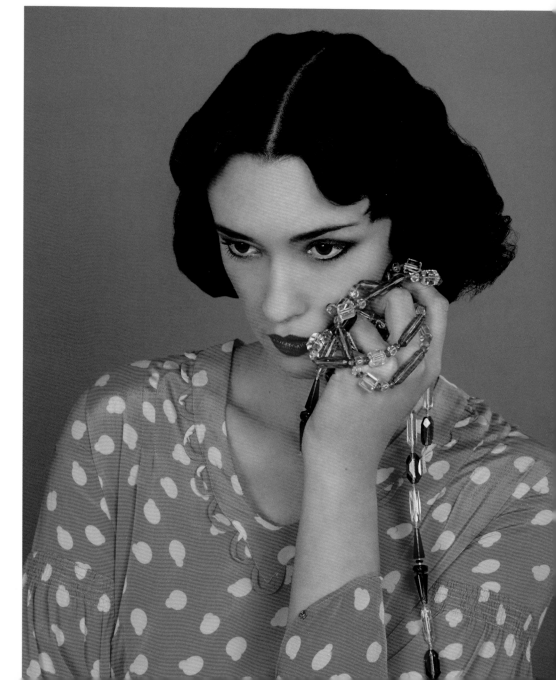

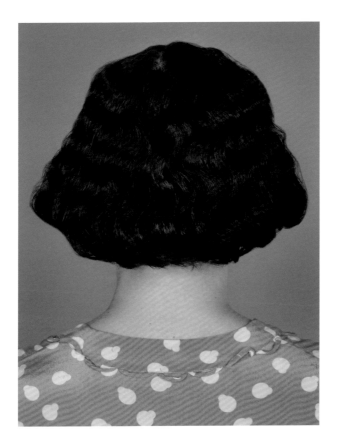

Make-up

For this look the make-up is the same as Look 3 (see page 34), but I created a shorter, sharper brow shape.

Hair

The hair is parted in the centre and then waved into a shorter bob using slightly bigger Marcel irons, which create a larger wave. Follow the same technique as shown on pages 29–31.

The fashionable smoky eye so popular in recent years has its origins in the smouldering looks of the 1920s.

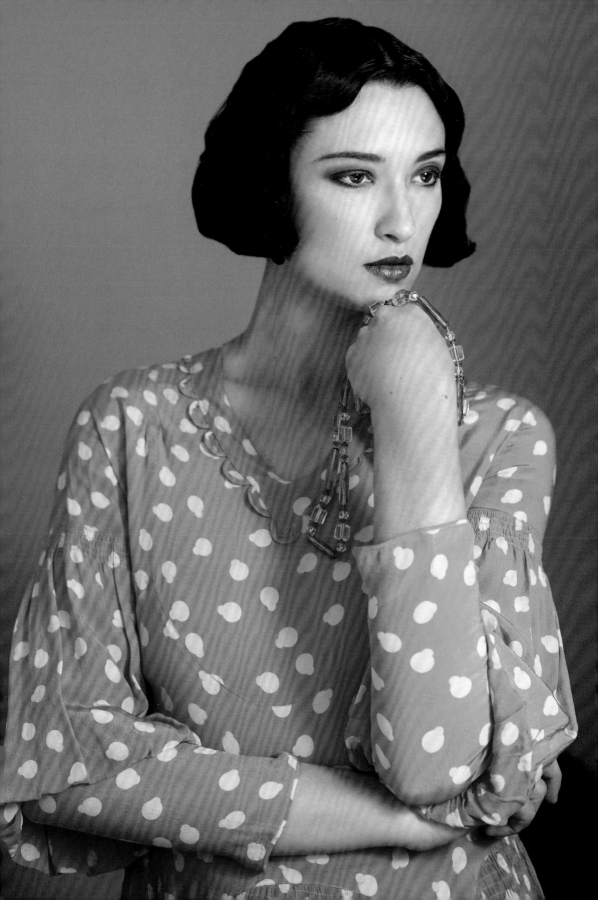

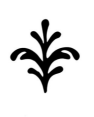

The 1930s

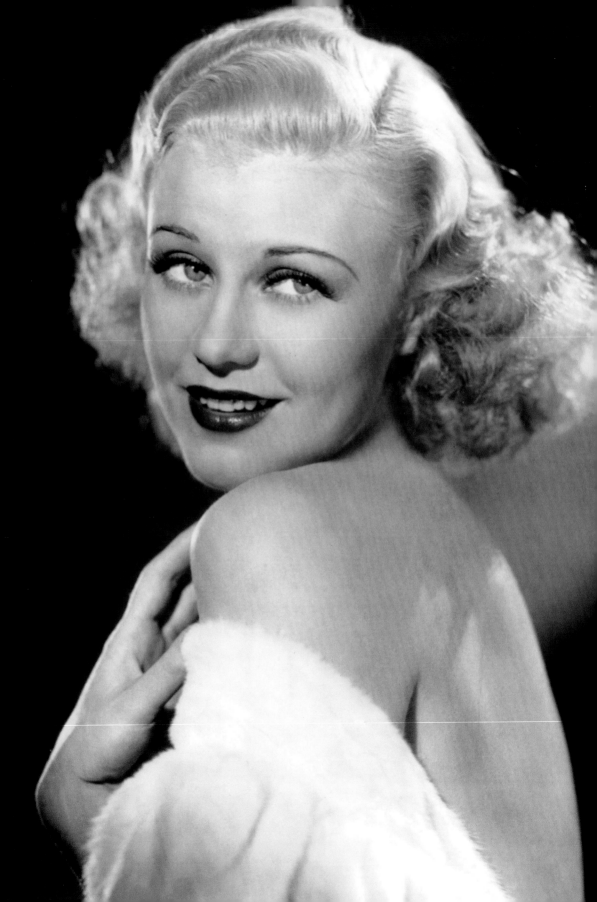

The 1930s

FOR ME, THE 1930S ARE THE EPITOME OF STYLE IN TERMS OF HAIR, CLOTHES AND MAKE-UP, AS THE SOMETIMES EXTREME LOOKS OF THE 1920S GAVE WAY TO AN UNRIVALLED ELEGANCE.

The glossy Hollywood films of the 1930s offered escapism to a population in the depths of a long economic depression. The economic downturn that began in the USA in 1929 soon affected the rest of the world, but as Britain and Continental Europe had not yet fully recovered from the First World War, the effect was not felt there as dramatically as it was in the USA, which in the 1920s had enjoyed a period of fun and excess – the Jazz Age. Despite this, cosmetics sales boomed on both sides of the Atlantic – evidence of the feel-good power of cosmetics and looking your best.

MAKE-UP

In the 1930s, lips were still made to look smaller, but without being forced into the unnatural, tiny bow shapes that were so fashionable in the 1920s. Lipsticks were available in more colours, with red, coral and raspberry being popular, while eyeshadows in blue, green, grey and brown were used in conjunction with blusher (or rouge, as it was known at the time) in vibrant coral and red. Thin, arched eyebrows were fashionable, as seen on stars such as Marlene Dietrich, Jean Harlow, Greta Garbo and Carole Lombard.

The use of cosmetics was well established, yet make-up was still manufactured using unregulated ingredients. This gave rise to a number of incidents of harmful ingredients causing health problems, skin damage and even blindness, leading to regulations being introduced in 1938.

Magazines showed women how to achieve the looks seen on their favourite actresses and celebrity endorsements were widespread, with major stars extolling the virtues of brands such as Max Factor, Coty and Maybelline. New products and formulations were introduced, with Helena Rubinstein laying claim to creating the first waterproof mascara in 1929. As in the 1920s, cosmetics compacts were things of beauty, being well designed and an essential part of every smart woman's outfit. Originally developed for the stars of the screen in 1935, Max Factor's Pan-Cake foundation was made widely available to the general public in 1938, as women's desire to emulate glamorous actresses continued.

Although, for the most part, being pale was still desirable, tanned skin become more fashionable, and powders in darker, sun-tanned shades appeared.

HAIR

The silhouette of the early and mid-1930s required hair to be short and close to the head. The Marcel wave was no longer as popular and, instead, perming, finger waving and pin curling were used. Some women wore short, waved fringes, others added hairpieces – called transformations – to lengthen a short style and create a different look. These chic, cropped styles complemented the elegant clothes of the era, and worked well with the hats and fur-collared coats that were in vogue.

Styles where the hair was slightly longer and fluffed out at the bottom appeared later in the decade and gave a softer, more glamorous look.

Opposite: Ginger Rogers, c.1935

Often beautifully packaged in enamel cases and combination compacts, the make-up products of the 1930s became fashion accessories, now that the use of make-up was something that women no longer felt they had to keep hidden. Popular brands were Maybelline, Max Factor, Du Barry, Dorothy Gray, Elizabeth Arden, Helena Rubinstein and Coty.

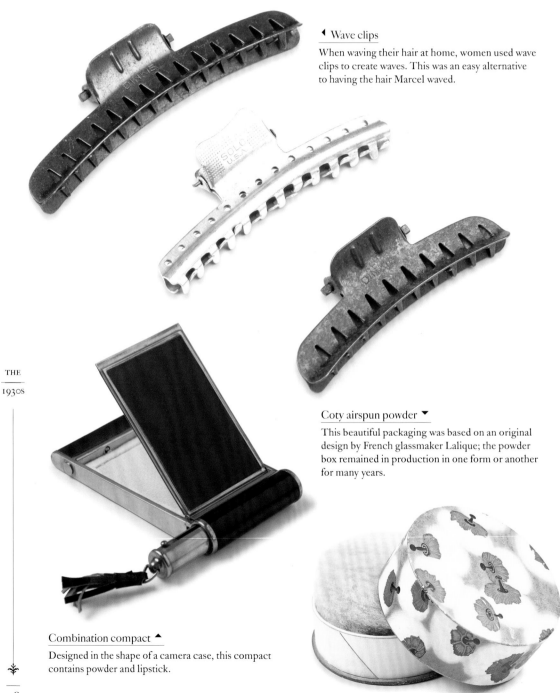

◀ Wave clips
When waving their hair at home, women used wave clips to create waves. This was an easy alternative to having the hair Marcel waved.

Coty airspun powder ▼
This beautiful packaging was based on an original design by French glassmaker Lalique; the powder box remained in production in one form or another for many years.

Combination compact ▲
Designed in the shape of a camera case, this compact contains powder and lipstick.

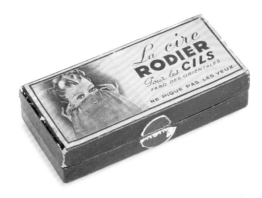

Ricil's cake mascara ▲

This type of solid mascara was activated by water – or more usually spit, which is why it was known for a long time as 'spit black'.

Rodier cake mascara ▲

In the 1930s mascara was available in blue, green, black, brown and purple. False lashes were also sold.

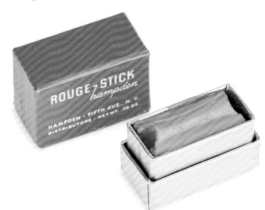

◄ Hampden rouge

Rouge was available in cream, paste and powder forms.

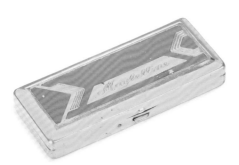

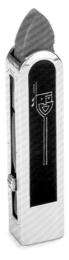

Maybelline cake mascara ▲

This cake mascara by Maybelline was packaged in a chic enamel case.

◄ ▲ Early 1930s lipsticks

The cosmetics containers of the time were small and neat – perfect for the streamlined clothes and bags of the era. The packaging of these lipsticks also reflects the clean lines and stylized decorations of the Art Deco period.

By the 1930s, cosmetics companies were offering rouge, powder and lipstick in a much broader choice of shades, as well as eyeshadows in blue, green, brown and purple. Magazines advised their readers to choose make-up to match their skin tones and clothes, rather than settling for one look for all, an approach that had led to some extreme looks in the previous decade. In the USA, the introduction of the 1938 Federal Food, Drug, and Cosmetic Act finally offered consumers protection from harmful, unregulated cosmetics.

A host of new make-up products and formulations appeared on the market in the 1930s.

LIPSTICK

In the 1930s the mouth was still made up to look smaller than it was, but in a more natural way than in the 1920s. Red, orange-red and raspberry were popular shades.

EYESHADOW

An array of coloured eyeshadows was available in the 1930s, from different shades of blue and violet to green and brown. These were often applied just to the lid but were sometimes taken right up to the eyebrows, and also under the eye on some looks. Lining pencils were also available in different colours.

BLUSHER

Sold in paste, cream and powder cake form, rouge came in shades from warm red and rose to the brightest raspberry. Rouge was worn high on the cheeks and, if colour was applied too liberally, a layer of powder would be used to tone it down. Some magazine articles at the time advised women on how to shape their faces through the placement of rouge, based on shading techniques used for films. Unless expertly done, however, this can look very odd.

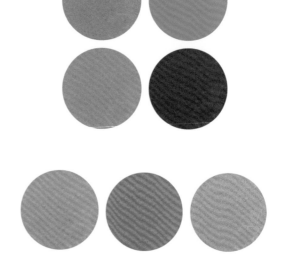

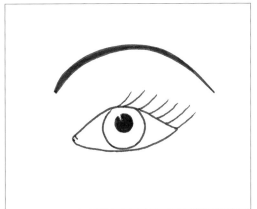

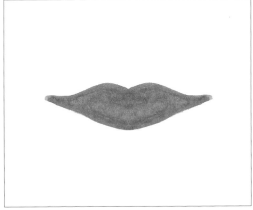

Brows

The very thin, neatly arched brow is one of the key elements of a 1930s make-up look. Arguably, the most famous exponent of this look was Marlene Dietrich, whose own brows were completely shaved off, rather than plucked into shape, and then pencilled in to perfection.

Lips

The desired mouth was a small rosebud shape but the lips were not as bee-stung as in the 1920s. Red continued to be the predominant lipstick colour.

With more colours available than ever before, women were increasingly encouraged by cosmetics advertising to experiment with their looks.

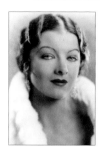

This is one of the most elegant, instantly recognizable looks of the decade. The reference image used here shows the actress Myrna Loy. For me, this style exudes 1930s Hollywood glamour and conjures up images of the stars arriving at their latest film premiere. The sleek lines of 1930s clothes complement the hair and make-up, and vice versa. Elements of this look, such as finger waves, have been adopted by the fashion world ever since.

THE

1930S

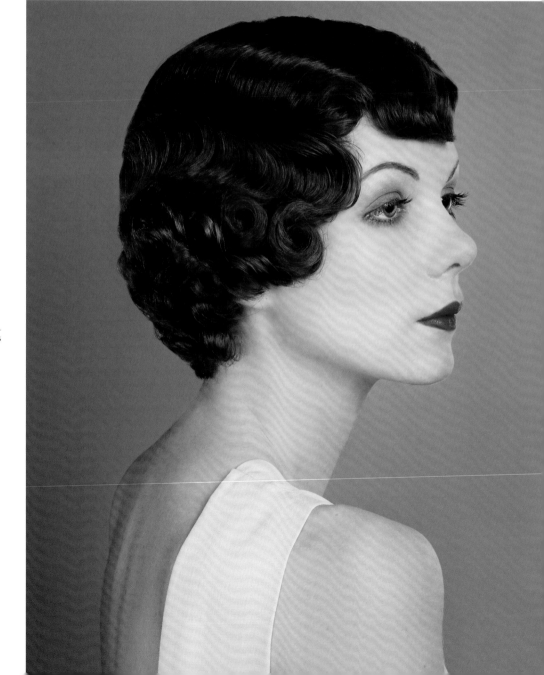

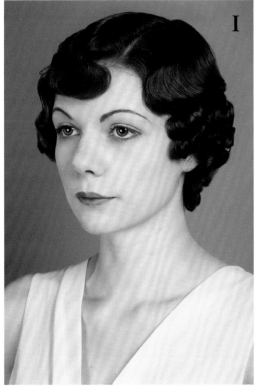

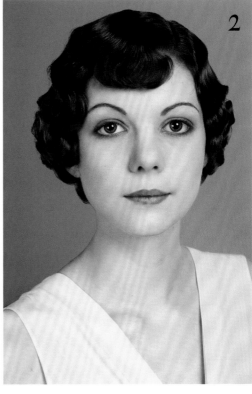

Step 1

Foundation: Apply foundation, followed by concealer and powder, as described in step 1 on page 19.

Step 2

Brows: The brows should be thin and shaped into a half-moon arch. I blocked out our model's full eyebrows using soap and camouflage cream (see the technique described in step 2 on page 27). Draw in the arch, using an angled brow brush with a wet tip to apply matte, dark shadow or brow powder. If you prefer, you can use a soft pencil.

Eyeshadow: Apply eyeshadow to the lid, blending it out at the socket line – I used a violet-coloured powder shadow with a matte texture. Take a little of this shadow under the bottom lashes at the outer corner of the eye, blending and fading it towards the inner corner.

Mascara: Coat the top and bottom lashes with black mascara. I didn't add false lashes, but at the time they were sometimes worn in the evening.

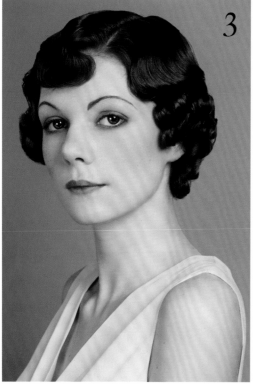

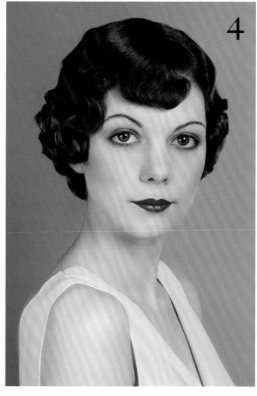

Step 3

Blusher: Apply blusher high up on the cheeks, quite near the eyes. Use a soft brush for this.

Step 4

Lipstick: To make the mouth appear smaller, first apply concealer or camouflage cream to block out the area you want to disappear, then powder over the top. This technique has to be done with great care to look effective and I would advise you not to make too dramatic a change as it will look strange. If you compare our model's natural lips (as seen above left) to the finished image (above), you can see the change in shape. To complete the look, apply raspberry lipstick with a brush.

This is a glamorous style that would have been done at the hair salon, and worn by a society lady in the 1930s.

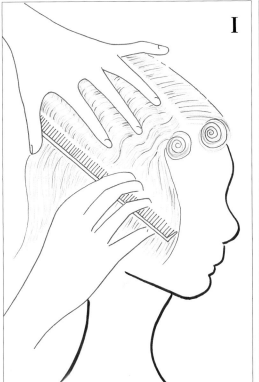

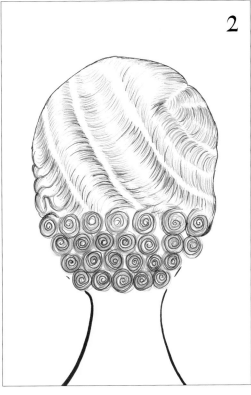

Step 1

Finger waves: The hair needs to be very wet. Place the forefinger on the hair, close to the parting, to hold the first wave in place. With your comb in the other hand, place it in the hair and push and slide the hair forwards, towards the face. With the comb still in the hair, holding it in place, lift the hand off the hair and move it down, placing the forefinger just below the wave. Next, comb the hair below the finger straight down, and push the hair to the opposite side to create the next wave. Move the hand down, as before, and repeat to create more waves, alternating the direction each time. You can secure the waves with an arc of sectioning pins, to hold them while pin curling. Do each side, then join the waves together at the back of the head, working towards the centre. In the illustration (above), the waves run at an angle, but a simpler version was done on our model, where the waves run down the head (see overleaf).

Step 2

Pin curls: Wrap a strand of hair around the forefinger to make the curl (see illustration below), then attach it firmly to the scalp with flat pins. The pin curls must sit just under the crest of the waves with each row alternating in direction – clockwise and anticlockwise. When the hair is completely dry, remove the pins, leaving the curls in place.

Finish with a fine mist of hair spray.

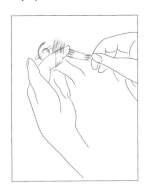

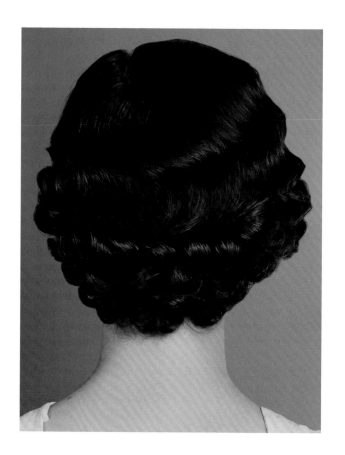

An elegant look that
encapsulates the glamour
of the 1930s.

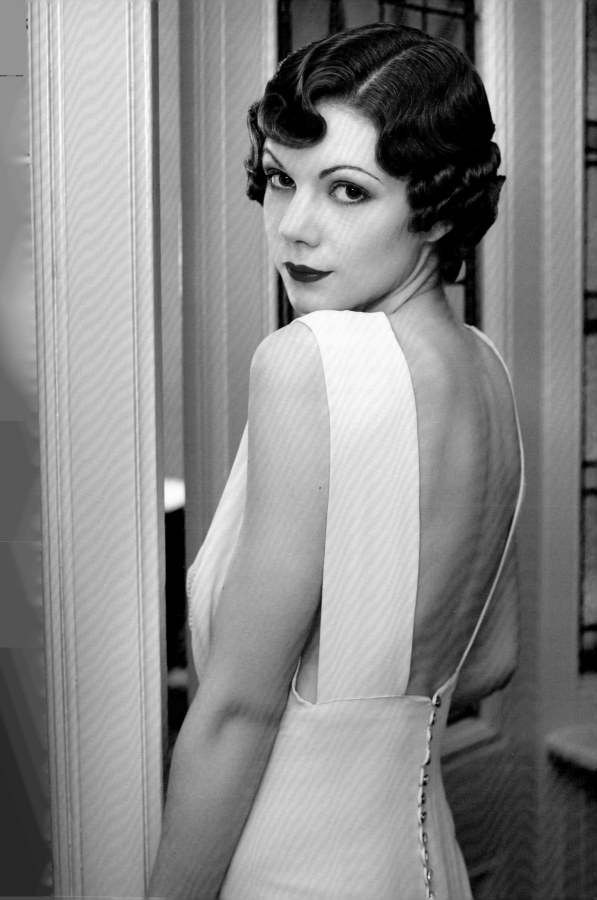

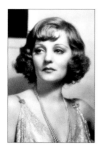

This style gives a slightly softer look than the more formal version shown on pages 52–7, using the same set. Here, the waves were combed out slightly to soften them, and the pin curls were flicked through for a fluffier style. In line with the fashion of the time, coats often had large collars, of either velvet or fur, and the hair was kept short so that the style wasn't ruined by rubbing against the coat. The crowns of hairstyles were kept flat, as hats were worn in the daytime. Our visual reference for this look is actress Tallulah Bankhead.

THE
1930S

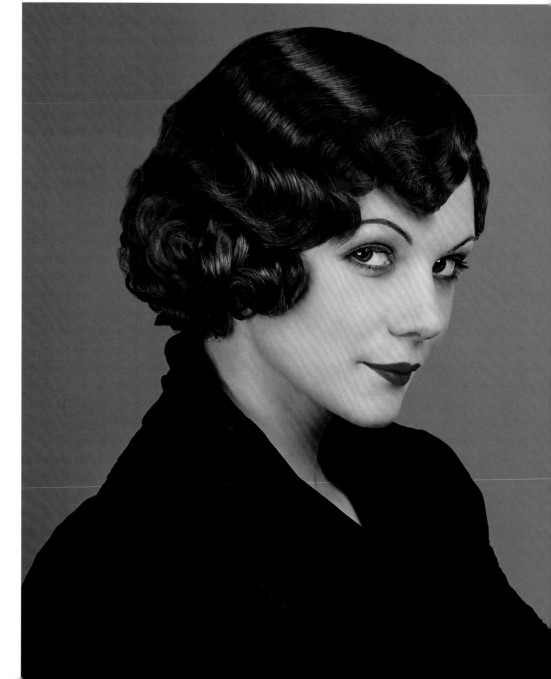

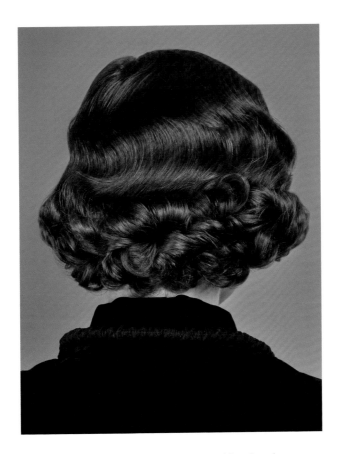

This hairstyle is a slightly softer variation of the one shown on pages 55–7, and would have been worn during the day or evening.

To capture the essence of an era, it is essential to get the shapes of the hair, eyebrows and lips right, as these visual reference points are the cornerstones of every look.

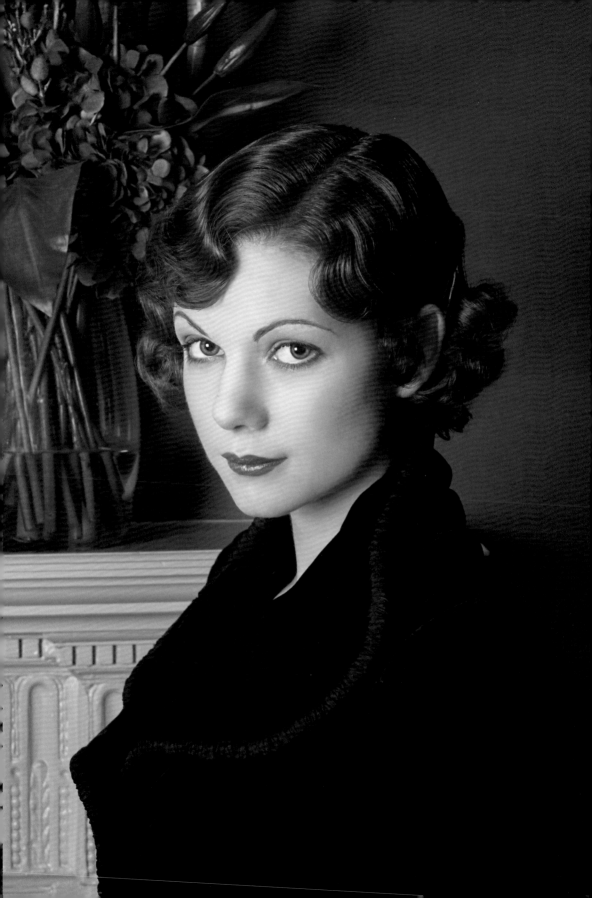

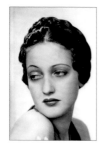

This look has been seen on many women in later decades and adaptations of it are still commonplace today. Popular in the late 1930s and into the 1940s, this style was worn by many screen icons, from Ginger Rogers to Dorothy Lamour, shown in our reference picture here. The make-up application is the same as for Look 1 (see pages 53–4), but I used a warm brown shadow on the eyes and a cake liner on the top lash line for emphasis.

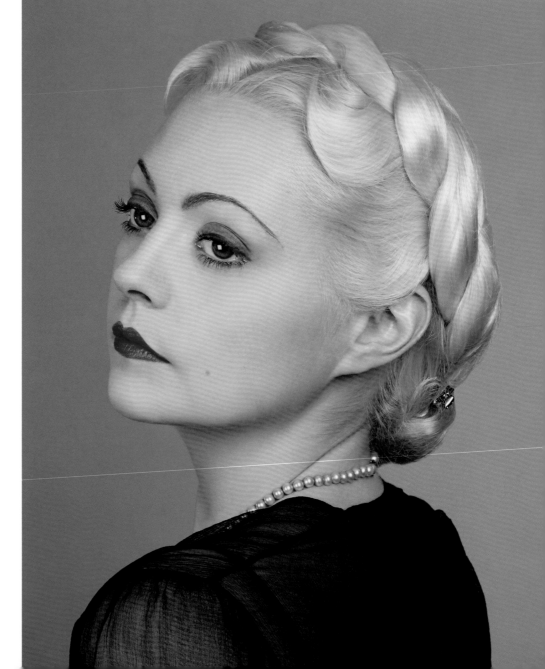

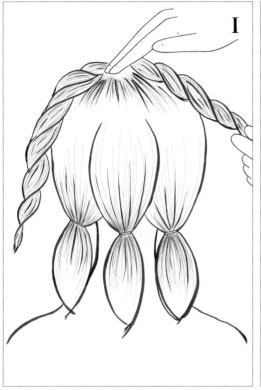

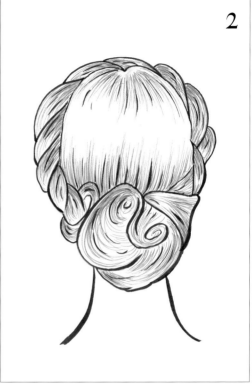

Step 1

A twisted hairpiece (switch) was used for this look, but it can easily be done with your own hair – just keep a section out from the back, and plait or twist and style it in the same way. You can also do this hairstyle using a modern hair extension.

Section the hair into three ponytails at the nape of the neck, as shown. Place the twisted hairpiece centrally on the top of the head and attach it firmly with a pin.

Step 2

Arrange the three ponytails together to form a low chignon and pin into place. Next, wrap the twisted hairpiece around the head and attach it at the base of the neck, using the ponytail bands to anchor the ends. Conceal any stray ends of hair by twisting them, tucking them in and securing with pins.

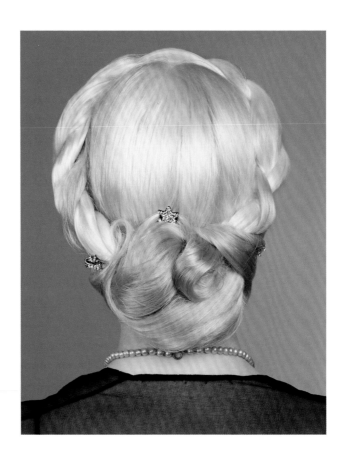

This glamorous style
has been finished with
small jewelled pins.

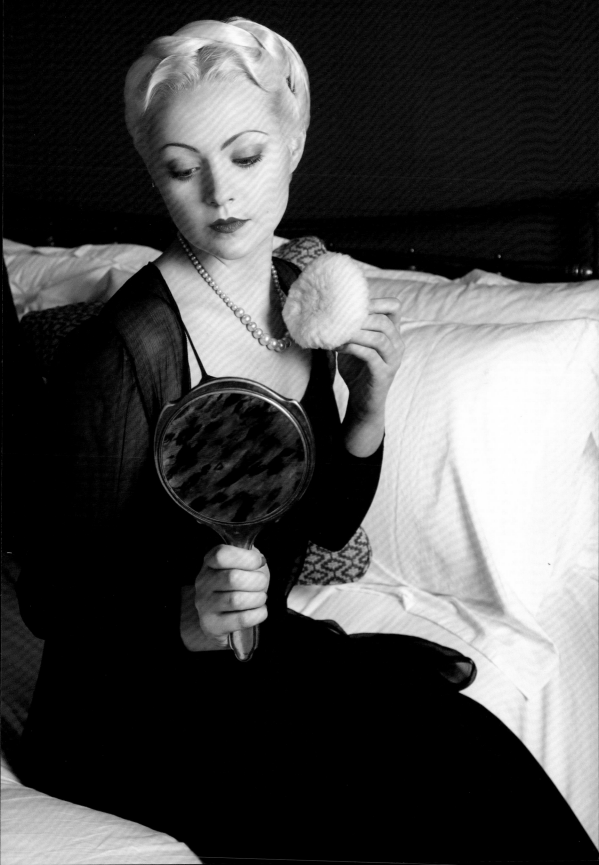

The 1940s

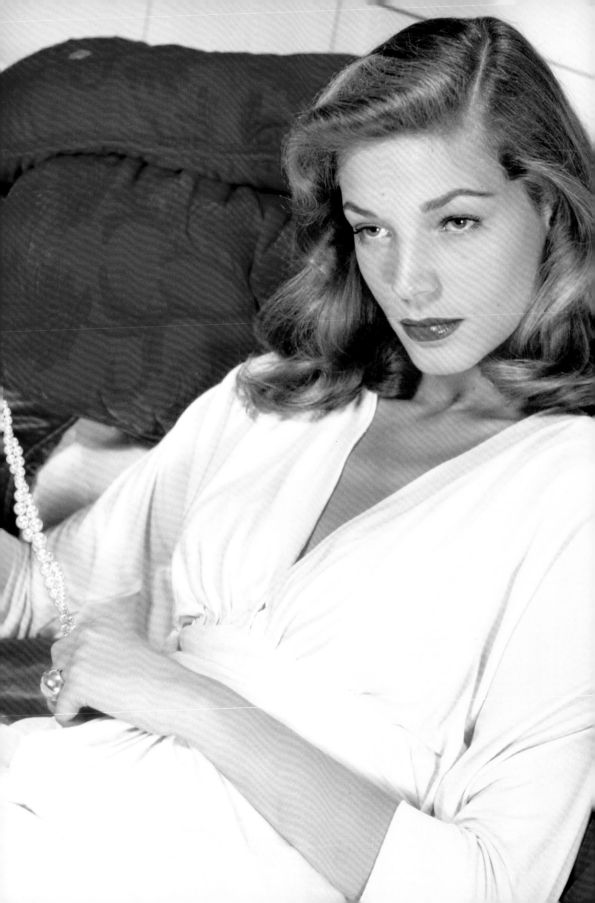

The 1940s

Cinema continued to provide escapism for a world at war, and looks from the silver screen inspired women's hairstyles and make-up. Actresses such as Rita Hayworth, Betty Grable, Gene Tierney, Ava Gardner and Veronica Lake were the style icons of the day, and photographer George Hurrell's images of these stars, among many others, are synonymous with Hollywood glamour.

MAKE-UP

Women were encouraged to wear make-up to boost morale and support the military. But, with some products hard to come by, they had to use home-made concoctions to attempt to replicate their idols' looks.

As well as facing restrictions in cosmetics' ingredients during the war, manufacturers were also forced to rethink their packaging because of shortages. Leading brands turned to paper and cardboard, rather than metal and plastic, and added text to their make-up boxes to reassure customers that the product inside was as good as ever.

During the 1940s, a smooth complexion was highly desirable. Clear skin, pencilled brows and full, red lips comprised the look of the decade, and new products made it easy to achieve.

Wearing make-up was considered to be such an intrinsic part of the war effort that powder compacts in the shape of army caps appeared, followed, in 1945, by celebratory victory compacts. After the Second World War, beauty products became more widely available again, although the UK was still subject to rationing into the early 1950s.

The cosmetics industry boomed during the war years, as it had done throughout the Great Depression of the previous decade. The importance of make-up as a morale-booster has become evident in subsequent economic crashes. In a response dubbed 'the lipstick effect', it seems that women turn to make-up in times of difficulty. I guess if we look good, we feel good.

HAIR

Practicality dictated hairstyles to a large extent during the war years. At times, more than 80 per cent of women were employed in factories, farms and other industries; hair had to be kept off the face and was often tied back for safety and ease of working.

Waved hair was the fashion and women used pin curls, perms or rags to achieve the fashionable looks of the day. Hollywood icons sported elaborate, glamorous styles, and although most women could not afford to visit a salon, they adopted these looks as best they could and styled their hair themselves along the lines of their icons.

Victory rolls, fringes and pompadours all featured in one form or another, and in this chapter Lou shows us how to create some of these styles. Women often added false fringes, curls and braids, as well as bulking out styles with 'rats', or nylon stockings filled with their own hair gathered from their hairbrushes. They decorated their hair with combs, ribbons and flowers. Hats were also often worn, so the crown of the hair was kept flat to accommodate them.

Opposite: Lauren Bacall, late 1940s

Two key things shaped the make-up of the 1940s: Hollywood and the Second World War. The morale-boosting effect that wearing make-up had on women was not lost on manufacturers, who produced cosmetics in patriotic-themed packaging, despite the shortages. Make-up products mainly consisted of powders, brow pencils, mascaras and lip colours. Popular brands of the decade include Max Factor, Tangee, Coty, Du Barry, Elizabeth Arden and Helena Rubinstein.

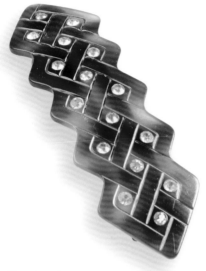

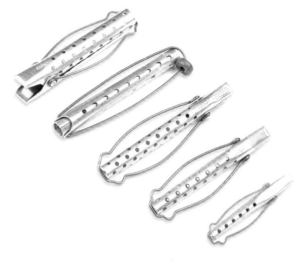

Hair slide ▲

Decorative hair slides, such as this glamorous example, were used to adorn various hairstyles of the 1940s.

Hair curlers ▲

Women used curlers like these at home, to curl the ends of their hair, and would often wear them to bed. They would sometimes resort to using makeshift curlers made out of stiff paper.

Max Factor Pan-Cake ▼

Originally made for screen stars, Max Factor's Pan-Cake became a bestseller when it was first released to the general public in the late 1930s. Easy to apply and with a long-lasting finish, it revolutionized the 1940s look, enabling women to achieve the flawless complexions of their favourite actresses.

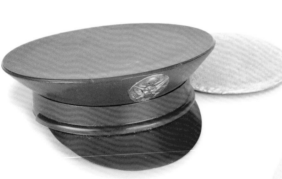

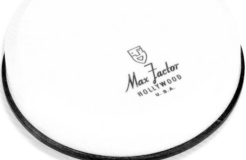

US Army powder ▲

Wearing make-up was seen as such an essential part of women's contribution to the war effort that various patriotic powder compacts, such as this one in the form of a peaked army cap, were produced.

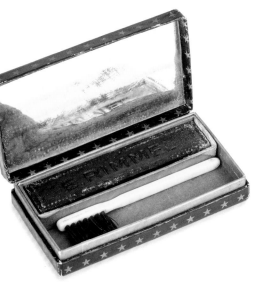

◀ Max Factor Pan-Stik

Launched in 1948, Pan-Stik was the forerunner of modern cream foundation formulas. Women could now carry their make-up base around with them, and the product was a huge success.

Rimmel mascara ▲

A staple of every woman's make-up, block mascara was activated by water and applied with a small brush.

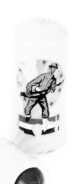

◀ US Army lipstick

Cosmetics companies started selling their products in patriotic packaging, such as this lipstick tube decorated with the image a soldier, to lift the spirits and support the war effort.

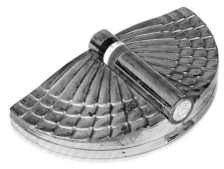

Flying colours compact ▲

This compact contains powder, rouge and lipstick.

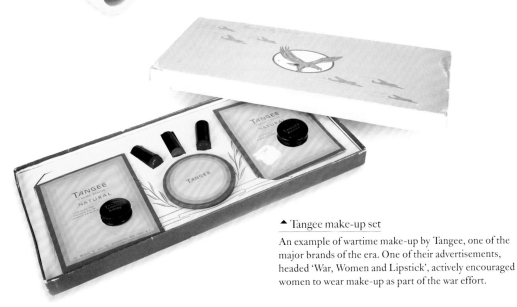

▲ Tangee make-up set

An example of wartime make-up by Tangee, one of the major brands of the era. One of their advertisements, headed 'War, Women and Lipstick', actively encouraged women to wear make-up as part of the war effort.

Along with a clear complexion and shaped brows, the cornerstone of 1940s make-up was a set of full, bright red lips. Aside from the lips, make-up colours were muted, with natural tones being the order of the day. Max Factor Pan-Cake foundation was very popular: activated with water, it gave a smooth, long-lasting finish, although it did make the complexion appear somewhat 'flat'. Remember that the eyeliner of the 1940s – if applied – was not flicked. Eyeliner flicks only came in the 1950s.

Many 1940s film stars kept the look designed for them by their studio throughout their careers.

LIPSTICK

All types of red were available at the time – cherry red, scarlet and orange red. Cosmetics companies frequently used Hollywood stars to promote their products. The advertisements of the time usually mentioned the stars' latest film release, and suggested that you too could look like a movie star if you wore the latest lip colour.

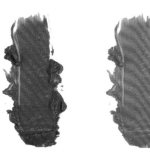 

EYESHADOW

Eyes were mostly kept natural: just cake mascara on the top lashes, brow pencil and perhaps some eye pencil to line the eyes. Eyeshadow, if worn, was grey or brown and used conservatively on the top lid. However, the eye make-up of movie stars, designed by the film studios, was more glamorous and involved a more extravagant use of shadow, although blue, grey and warm brown continued to be the most popular shades.

BLUSHER

Still known as rouge at the time, blusher was available in both cream and powder form. Coral, soft raspberry and rose tones were used, but only sparingly.

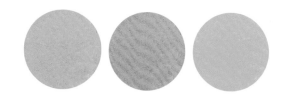

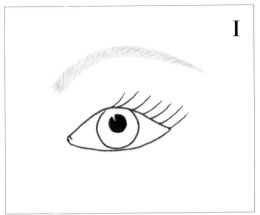

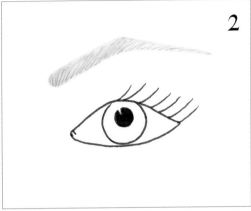

Brows Look 1

Eyebrows were an important feature, and many of the era's film stars sported strong brows with heavily coloured-in arches. However, numerous women wore a softer version of this look and the predominant shape was a more natural, gentle arch.

Brows Look 2

The sharply angled classic 1940s brow, as seen on actress Lauren Bacall (see page 68).

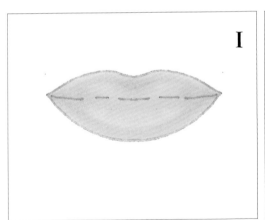

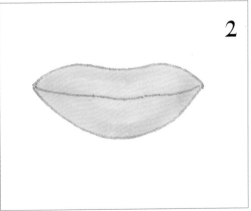

Lips Look 1

When recreating a 1940s look, it is important to get the lip shape right – full, rounded lips were the look of the decade. Overdrawn lips are plain to see in the photographs of many stars of the era, such as Lucille Ball, but they are hard to maintain in real life.

Lips Look 2

Made famous by Joan Crawford, this more dramatic lip shape – dubbed the Hunter's Bow lip or the Smear – was also popular. The centre of the top lip has just a slight dip, and the mouth is drawn almost into a snarl.

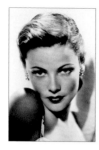

The classic 1940s make-up look is probably one of the most instantly recognizable, and it can seem just as fresh and glamorous today as it did during that iconic decade. It was actually quite a simple look compared to those of other eras and it is easy to adapt a typical daytime make-up look, as worn every day by young women at the time, to create a more glamorous evening version, or even one fitting for a bride. With interpretations of it frequently seen at red-carpet events today, this elegant make-up look has stood the test of time and suits women of all ages. Our reference picture is of Gene Tierney.

THE

1940S

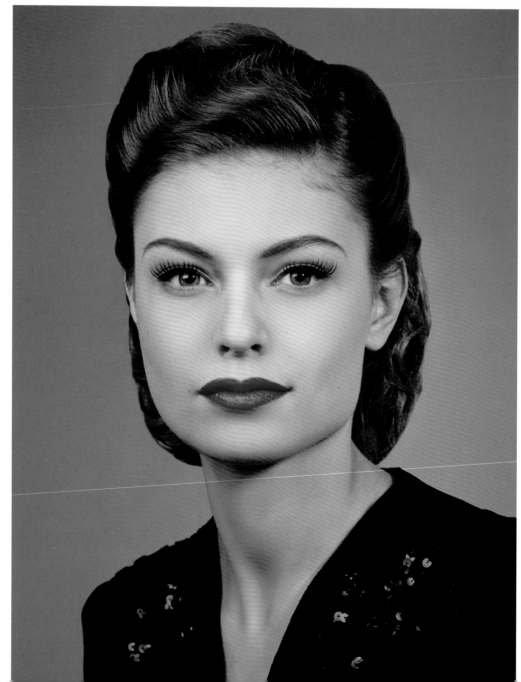

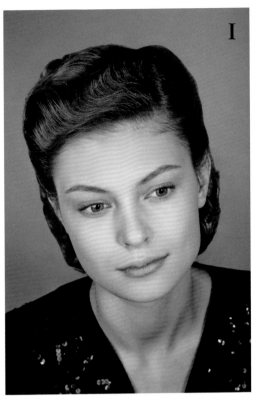

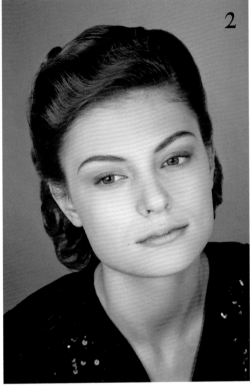

Step 1

Foundation: Apply foundation, followed by concealer and powder, as described in step 1 on page 19.

Step 2

Brows: Use an angled brush and a matte eyeshadow or brow powder to colour in and shape the eyebrows. The shape of the brows is important (see page 73), and the ideal was a natural, rounded arch, rather than an extreme arch.

Eyeshadow: Using a tapered shadow brush, apply a matte, soft, mid-brown powder shadow to the lid and blend. On some evening looks, the shadow was taken a little higher up towards the eyebrow and blended, with different shades being used (see page 72 for a colour reference guide).

Mascara: Apply dark brown mascara to the top lashes only. I used cake mascara for this look.

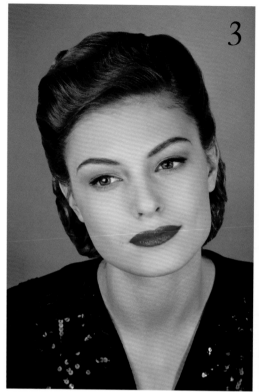

3

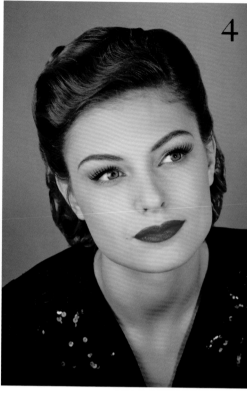

4

Step 3

Eyeliner: Apply eyeliner to define the top lid. I used a cake liner in dark brown. Keep it close to the upper lash line and don't flick it out at the corners. Eyeliner was not always applied; when it was, pencils were sometimes used, but it was never flicked out at the corners – flicks belong in the 1950s.

Blusher: Apply blusher in a coral shade to the apples of the cheeks and blend it out onto the cheekbones, using a soft brush, to give the face warmth and shape.

Lipstick: An essential for a 1940s look, lipstick came in various shades of red and was worn by all ages. The shape is important (see page 73), with the top lip slightly overdrawn and rounding from the outer corners to give a full appearance. Use a pencil in the same shade as the lipstick to draw the outline, then fill in with lipstick using a brush.

Step 4

Lashes: If you would like to achieve a more glamorous Hollywood or evening look, you can add full false lashes, as I did here. Make sure to keep them close to the lash line.

With a few tweaks, the basic set shown opposite can be made into a whole range of glamorous 1940s hairstyles (see pages 78–89).

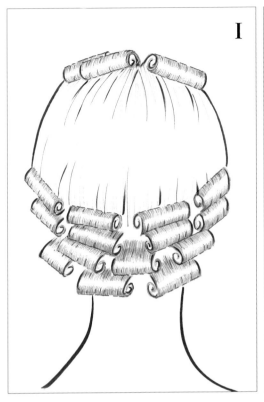

1

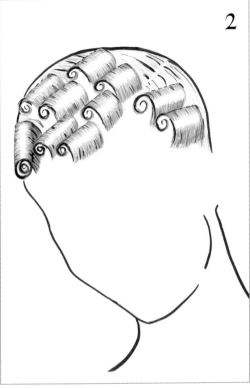

2

Step 1

Set the hair in the direction you want the waves to go. This may sound obvious, but the key to the success of the style is the set being correct in the first place. The crown of the head is kept flat and medium rollers (2cm/¾ inch) are placed in a curved horseshoe shape around the base of the head. (Pin curls would have been used at the time for many styles, but we use heated rollers now.)

Set the front and side rollers, as shown above right. Spray setting lotion on each section of hair before rolling. The side rollers go up and slightly back at an angle away from the face. The front-to-side rollers are slightly angled to blend in with the sides. Make sure all the ends are rolled in neatly, otherwise they will not give a smooth look when the hair is brushed out. Remove the rollers when they are cool.

Step 2

To style the wave at the front, brush through the front section, push the hair forward and the wave should form automatically. The hair can then be pinned into position and the back styled as required (see variations on the following pages). If the hair is very long, a fine net or a snood can be used to shorten the back without using grips.

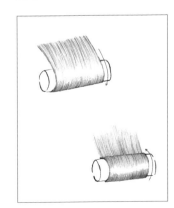

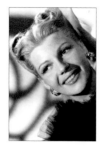

This look is a variation on Look 1 (see pages 74–7). The hair has been styled into the classic 1940s rolls at the front and a glamorous twist at the back. This would have been an evening hairstyle in the 1940s, and seven decades later, it would look just as stunning at any formal occasion. Our reference is the beautiful actress and dancer Rita Hayworth, who starred in musicals opposite Gene Kelly and Fred Astaire, but is probably best known for playing a glamorous *femme fatale* in the 1946 film *Gilda*.

THE

1940S

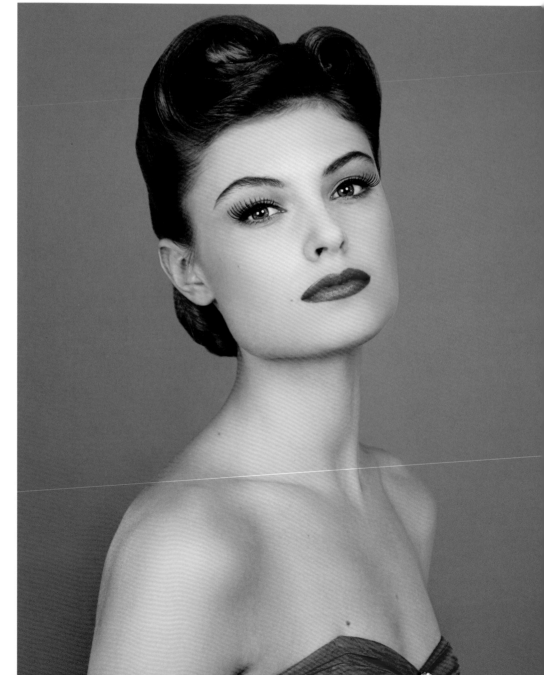

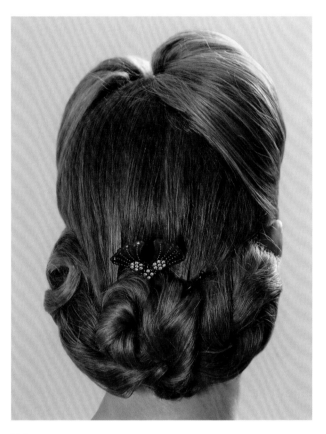

Hair

Start by setting the hair as shown in step 1 on page 77. To style the hair at the front into rolls, take a section of hair at one side to make the first roll. Backcomb it lightly and smooth the surface. Keeping one hand on the scalp, wrap the section of hair around your hand and make it into a roll. Pull this forward on the head, so that the front of the roll is open and the back is closed. Secure with pins inside the roll so they do not show.

Make a second roll on the other side and pin it in place as before.

To style the hair at the back, divide it into three sections and twist each one into the required style, starting with the sides and doing the central section last. Secure each section with grips, tucking them in well so they can't be seen.

The back of the hair is decorated with an ornate 1940s hair clip.

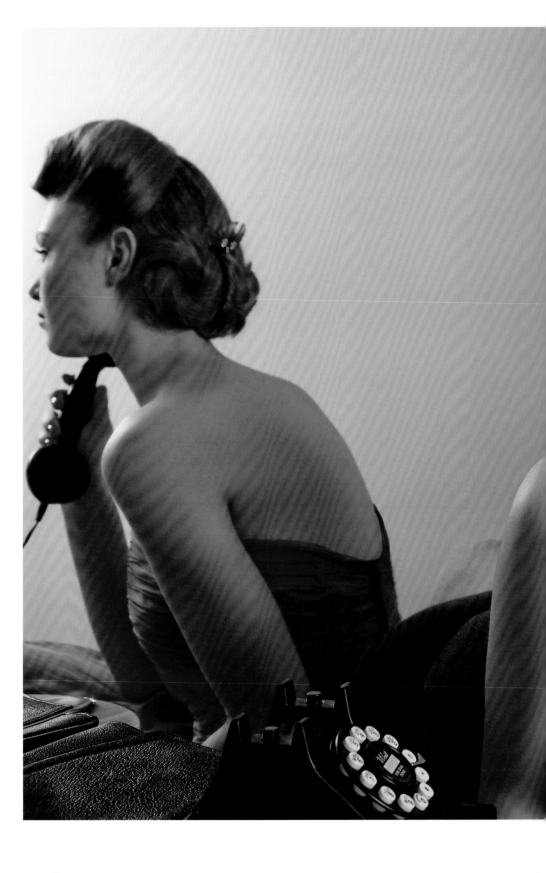

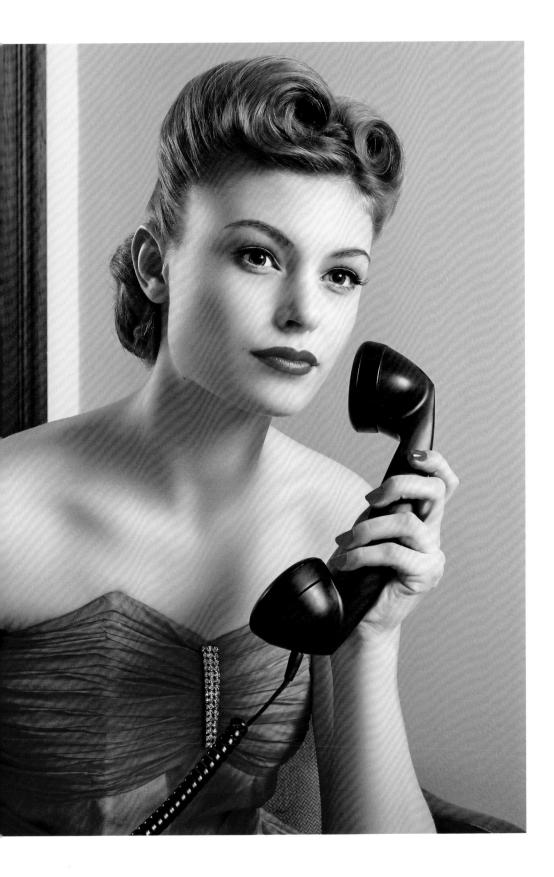

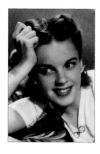

The make-up here is the same as for Look 1 (see pages 75–6), but the lips are a slightly deeper, cherry red. This hairstyle, based on the same set as in Look 1, has quite a simple front, with sections of hair taken on either side of the parting and styled on the crown of the head. The back is more ornate, and as the model's hair was quite long, Lou shortened it after removing the curlers by taking some of the length and using grips to secure it close to the head. The ends were then styled into small curls and pinned in place. The hair is finished with a 1940s slide. Our reference image is of actress Judy Garland.

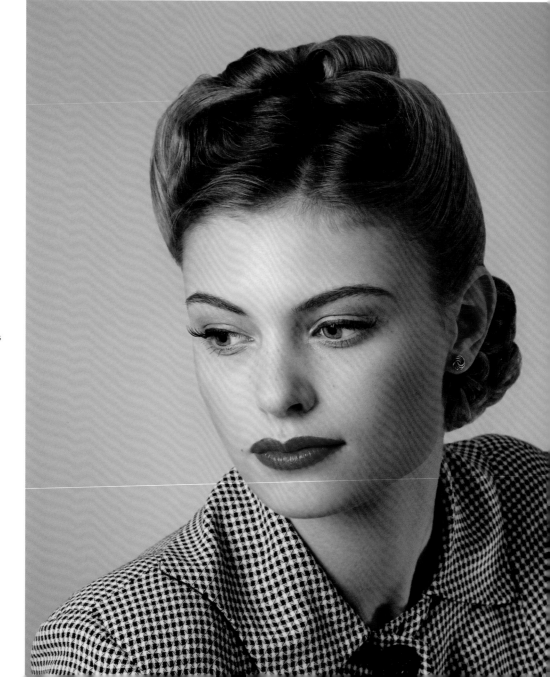

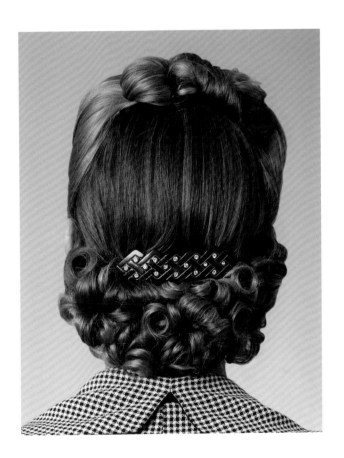

In the 1940s, cake mascara
would sometimes double up
as eyeliner, giving a watery,
non-solid line.

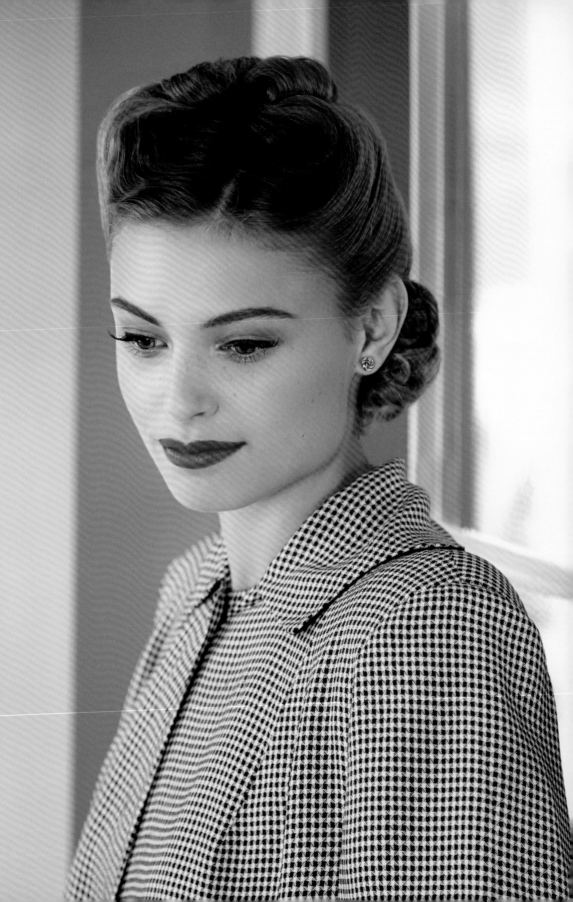

The lipsticks of the 1940s
were mostly matte, so a dab
of Vaseline could be applied
to give a shiny finish, if desired.

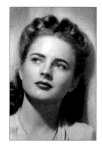

This look features a simple type of hairstyle that would have been worn by many women as it is easier to do on oneself. Our reference image shows the actress Coleen Gray. Having set the hair as shown on page 77, the sides were clipped up on top of the head with the back left loose and the length lightly shaken through to fluff out the curls. The make-up features shaped and coloured brows, soft eyeliner and brown eyeshadow, minimal mascara on the top lashes only, a touch of blusher and lip colour. For a simpler look, just focus on getting the brow and lip shapes right (see page 73), and then add mascara.

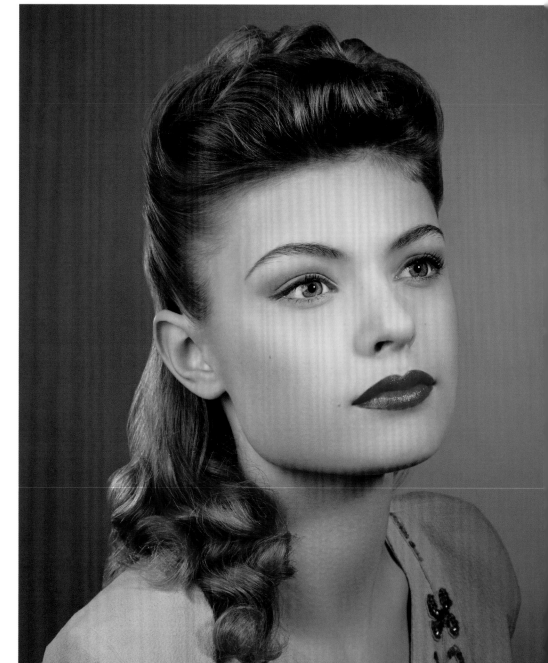

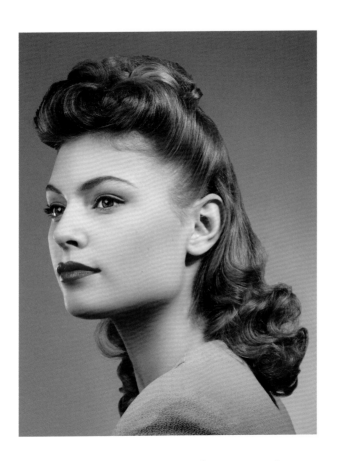

Women working in wartime
factories kept things simple, often
wearing only powder and lipstick.
Hair was styled off the face or
wrapped in a scarf for practicality.

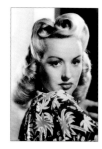

This classic 1940s look features large rolls on the forehead, as worn by actress Betty Grable in our reference image. This is a clean, stylish hairdo, kept in place at the back with a hair slide. These rolls have been styled in the same way as in Look 2 (see page 79), just made a little higher with some more backcombing. Many women in the 1940s had dry hair as a result of using perming solutions, detergent shampoos and lacquer, which was needed to hold some styles in place, so brilliantine was applied to smooth the locks and add shine. Today we can use a little serum where needed.

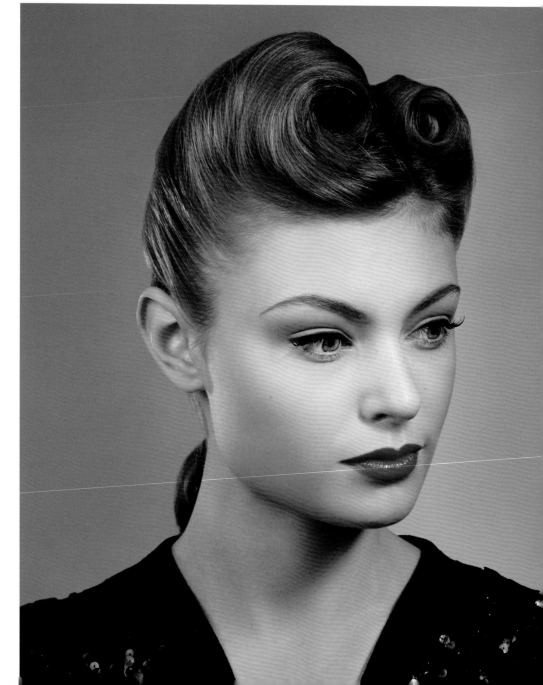

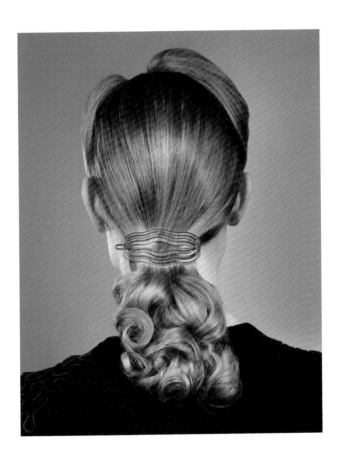

Blusher was used sparingly in the 1940s – the emphasis was on the lips and the brows.

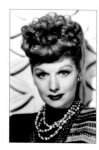

An instantly recognizable look, this hairstyle was most notably worn by blonde bombshell Betty Grable and famous redhead Lucille Ball (pictured here). The important thing to remember about this style is that the curls should sit towards the front of the head and fall forward on to the forehead. The make-up is a glamorous, standard 1940s look, as in Look 1 (see pages 75–6), but I applied some red-rust eyeshadow to the brows to match the model's hair colour. The lips are slightly overdrawn to achieve the ideal shape (see page 73). If you use eyeliner on the upper lash line, as I have, remember not to flick it out at the corners.

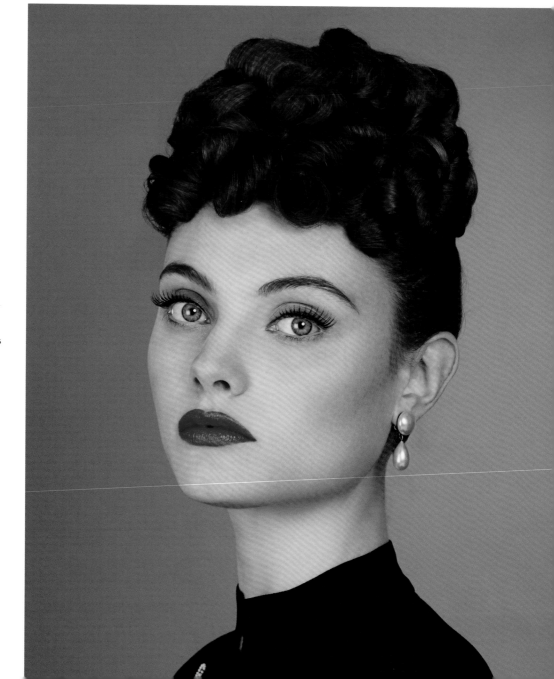

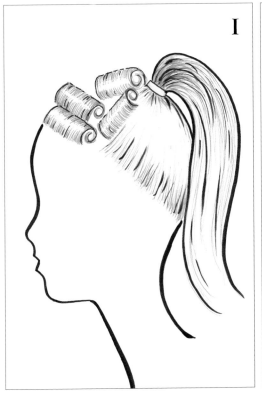

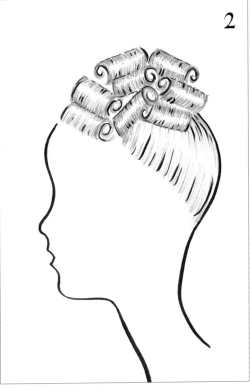

Step 1

Choose the size of rollers you want to use to set the hair according to the size of curls you want for the finished style: the larger the rollers, the bigger the curls will be. Here, we used medium-sized rollers (2cm/¾ inch) on the model's medium-length hair.

Section off the front of the hair and brush the rest into a high ponytail on the crown of the head. For more control of a lot of hair, you can section the back into two ponytails. Lou used the cross-grip technique (where grips are crossed over each other in an X shape) to take the hair up at the back, but a hairband will give more control if you are not used to doing this style.

Set the front section of the hair on medium-sized heated rollers, placing them in a random way.

Step 2

Set the hair in the ponytail in the same way.

When the rollers have cooled, remove them. Comb the hair on to the top of the head, brushing it towards the centre to narrow the back, but not making a pleat. Arrange the curls, making sure the hairband is hidden, and pin them in place.

Add two combs in the back, below the curls, both for decoration and to hold the hair more securely.

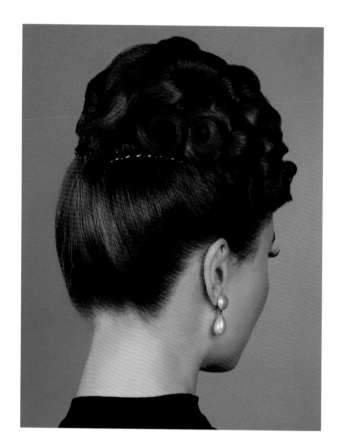

Combs, slides and other hair
accessories were widely used in the
1940s to add visual interest and
keep styles firmly in place.

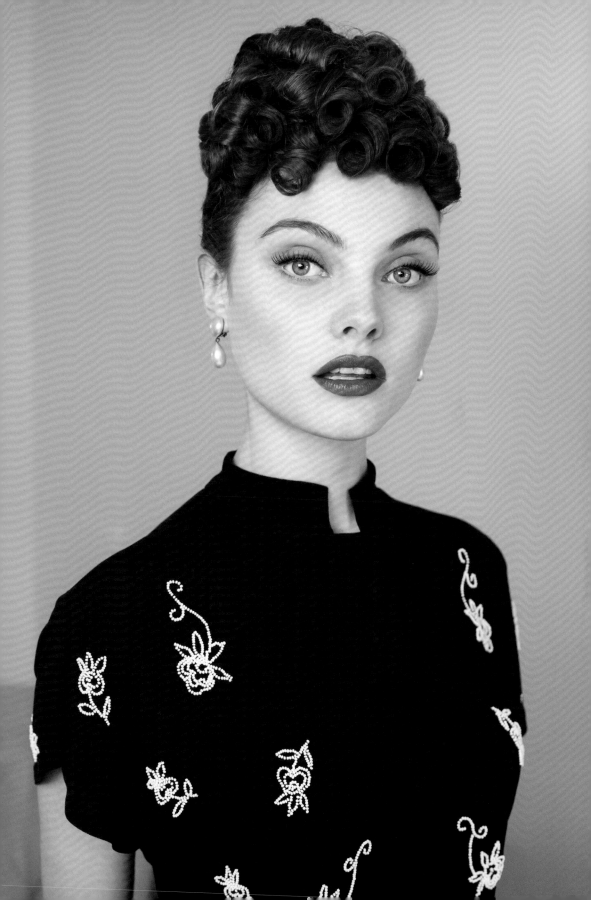

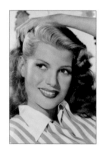

This is a simpler hairstyle that can be achieved on shoulder-length hair to give the 1940s look. Our reference picture shows Rita Hayworth. Her fellow Hollywood star Veronica Lake was famous for her peekaboo hairstyle, and her long, large-waved pageboy style that fell over one eye was widely copied. It was also considered a safety hazard in the workplace, with a number of women wearing the style getting their hair caught in machinery. Veronica made a public information film showing her hair being styled and pinned off the face, and urged women to do the same for safety's sake.

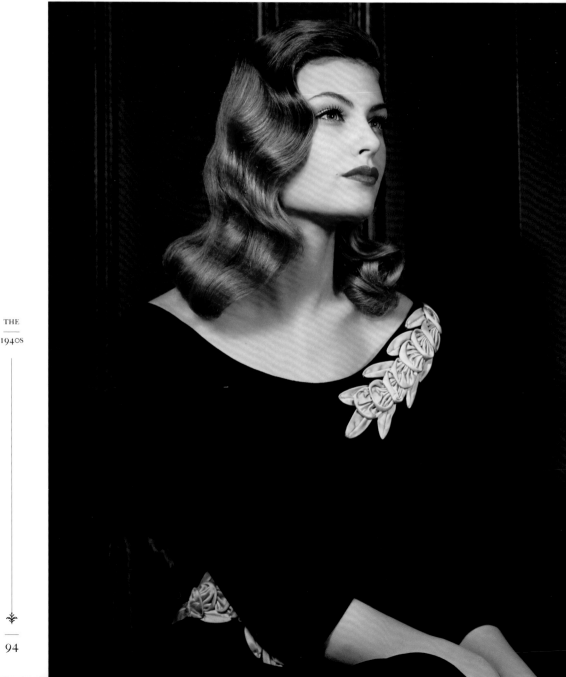

THE

1940S

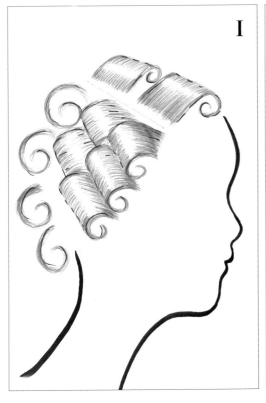

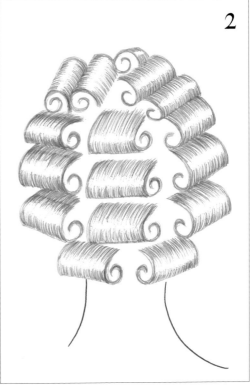

Step 1

Choose the roller size depending on the size of waves you would like.

Create a side parting, then set the hair in heated rollers, as shown, making sure the rollers are angled in the correct direction. Start with sides and roll the hair under, tucking the ends in neatly. Spray setting lotion on each section of hair before rolling.

Step 2

Set the back section of the hair in the same way.

The set shown here, with rollers starting at the top of the head and running all the way down, will give waves in the crown area of the hair, but the finished style should only have natural lift, not too much height, at the crown.

When the rollers have cooled, remove them and brush the hair into soft waves, making sure the crown is smoothed down.

To add shine and remove any flyaway hairs, apply a little serum with the palms of the hands, smoothing them over the waves.

This style can be clipped up at one side or both for variations and was a very popular look.

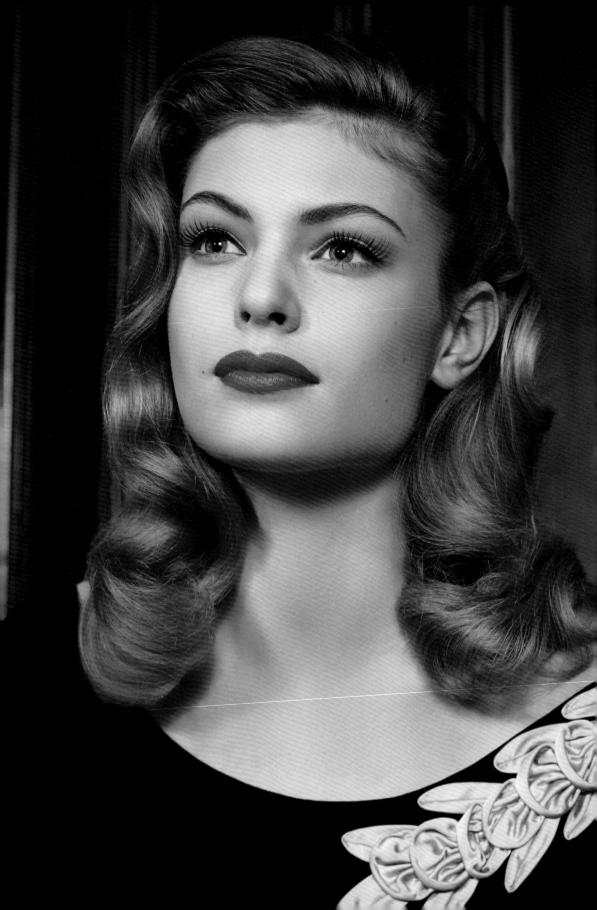

In the 1940s, this style would have been achieved with reverse pin curls set just around the edges of the hair.

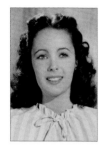

This is a more youthful, simple look, which was widely worn by women in the 1940s, as seen here on a young Elizabeth Taylor. Having achieved early fame through the starring role in *National Velvet* at the age of 12, Elizabeth appeared in full make-up on screen and at premieres by the time she was 15. Hollywood studios required their stars to keep up the image that had been created for them at all times, and Elizabeth went on to become known as one of the film industry's greatest beauties. The make-up here is the same as in Look 1, but with smaller false lashes.

THE
—
1940S

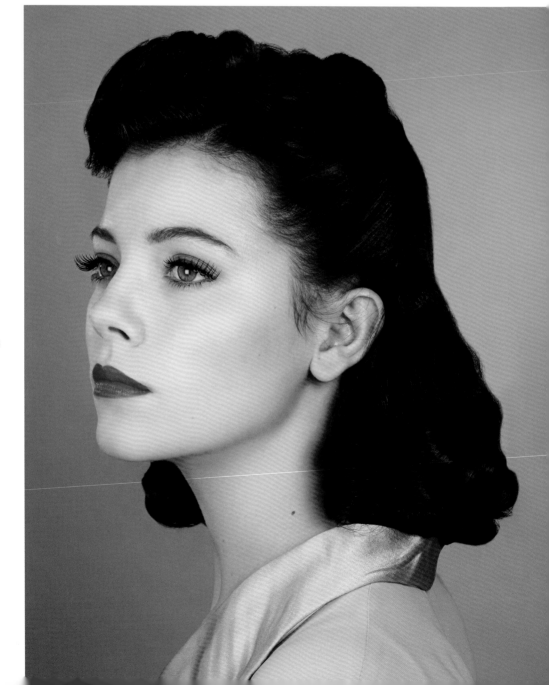

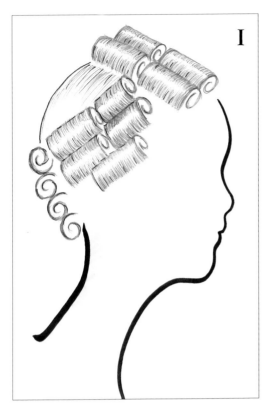

Step 1

Set the hair, as shown above, using heated rollers or hot sticks (bendy rollers). Spray setting lotion on each section of hair before rolling.

When the rollers have cooled, remove them and brush the hair through.

Take up the hair on each side of the parting in turn, style it into a roll and secure with pins, as described on page 79.

Leave the back section down in loose waves.

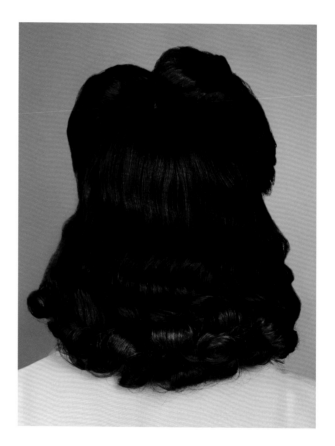

This is make-up fit for a 1940s starlet. A normal girl would have worn a simpler look, with no false lashes or eyeliner, just lip colour.

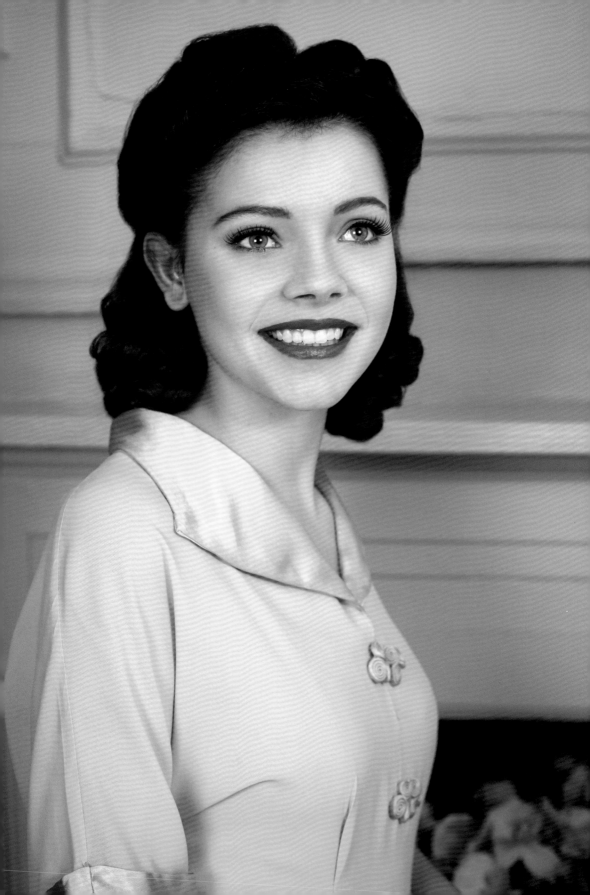

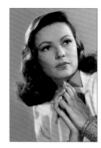

Another variation on a classic 1940s hairstyle that would look at home on the red carpet today. Our reference image is of Gene Tierney, one of the most beautiful Hollywood actresses of the era. The hair was set from a left side parting with heated rollers, as shown on page 95, and then styled into soft waves with a smooth crown. To smooth the hair, put a little serum in the palm of your hand and stroke it onto the hair, then comb through. This style sounds simple, but the success of all of these hairstyles depends on the set being done accurately in the first place.

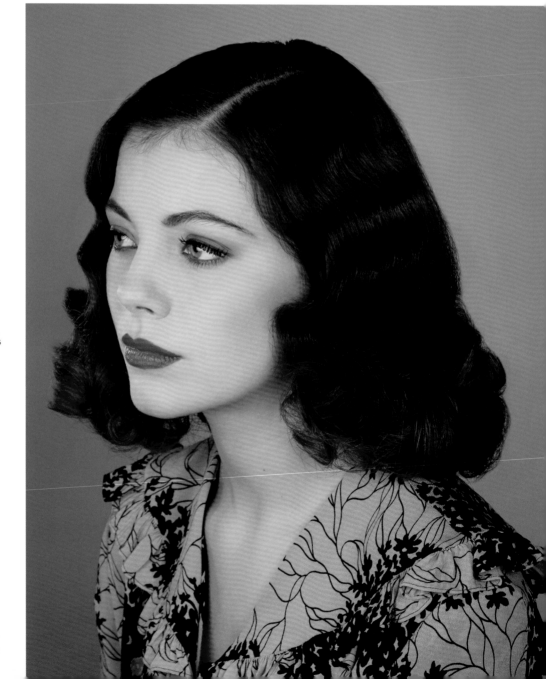

THE

1940S

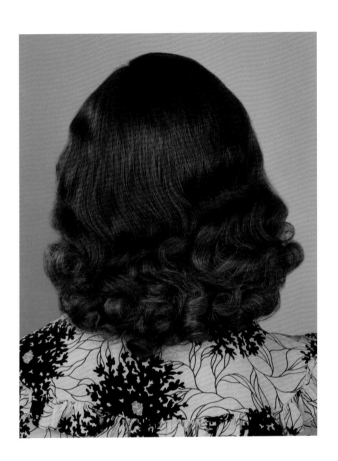

When rouge became
difficult to obtain during
the war, women often used
lipstick to add a little colour
to their cheeks.

One of the easier looks of
this era to style, this is a
versatile hairstyle that can be
clipped up at the side.

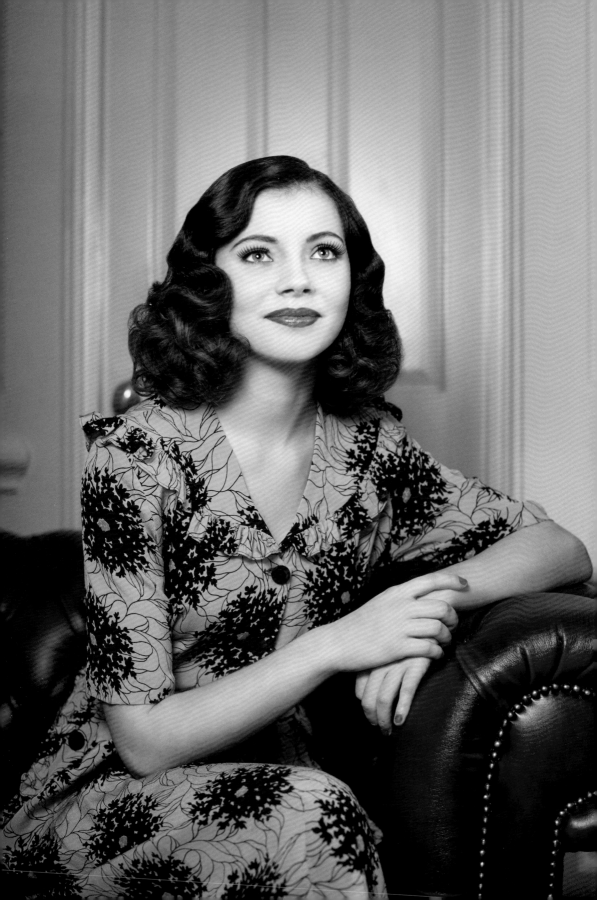

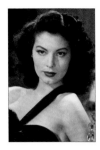

This stunning look is one of my favourites. Worn by Hollywood stars such as Rita Hayworth and Ava Gardner (pictured), this is a fluffier version of the waved shoulder-length styles of Looks 7 and 9 (see pages 94 and 102). In the 1940s, the hair would have been curled at home with small reverse pin curls or by setting it on tiny curlers like those pictured on page 70. Lou styled the hair by setting it in the same way as shown on page 95 using hot sticks (bendy rollers) and then brushing it through afterwards.

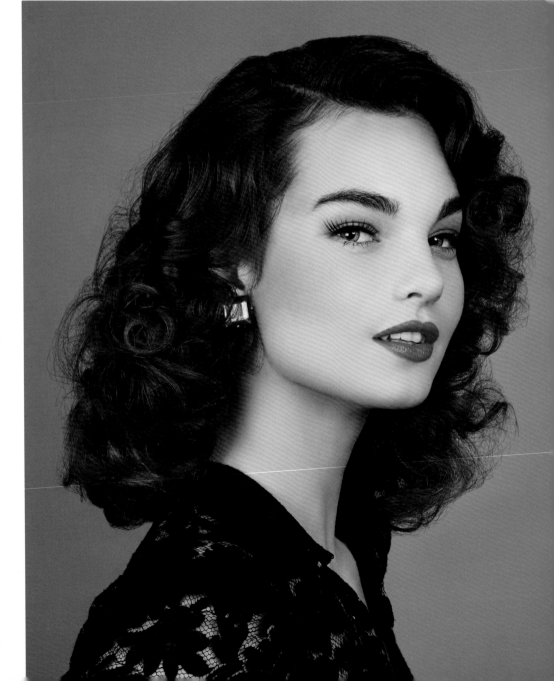

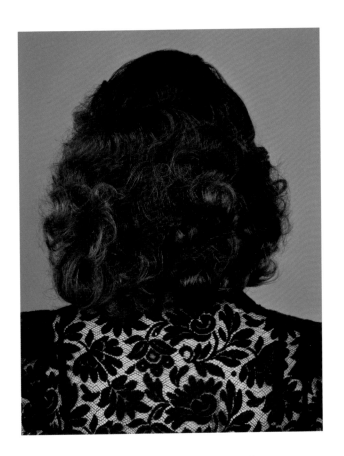

Shoulder-length hair is
ideal for a wide variety of
styles from the 1940s.

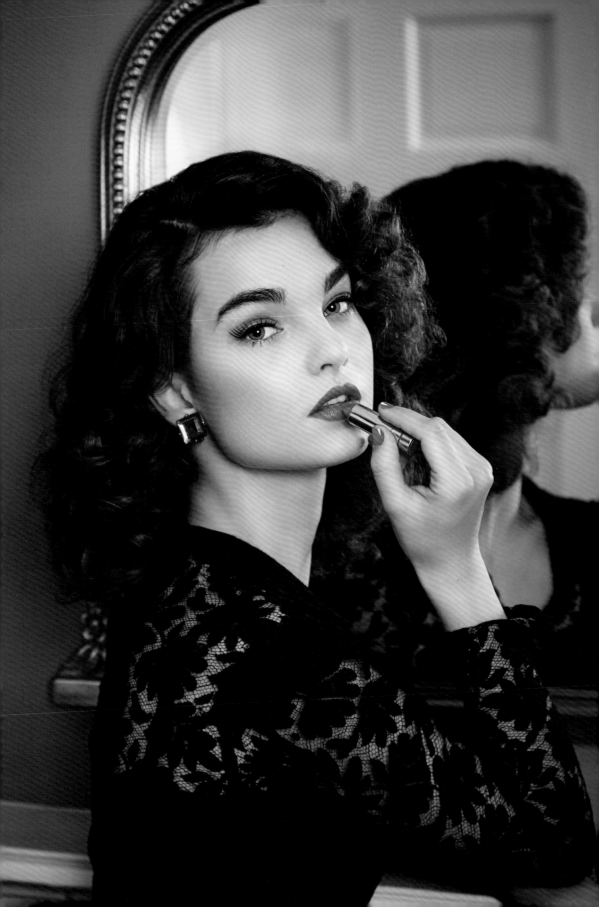

Long false lashes add a touch
of glamour, while the brows have
been left naturally full. A classic
bright red lip completes the look.

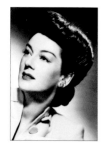

This hairstyle features a large fringe, as seen in our reference image of actress Rosalind Russell. Many variations of this style were worn, from sleek and simple versions suitable for every day to dramatic, over-the-top creations. Women would sometimes use a false fringe to achieve this look but you can use your own hair, as Lou did on our model.

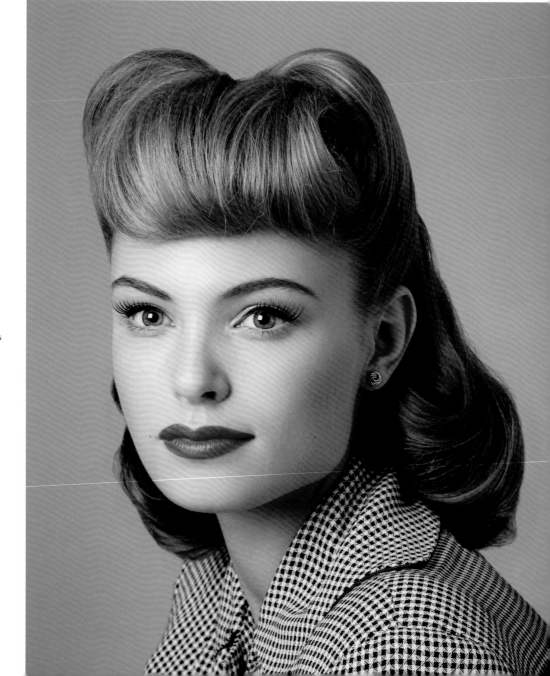

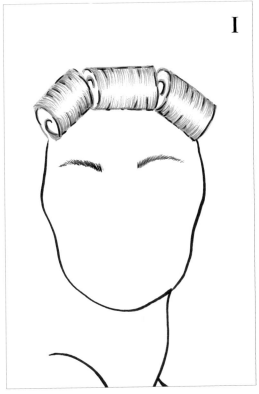

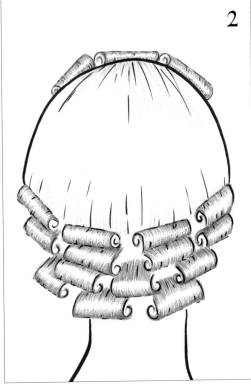

Step 1

Set the hair, as shown above, using heated rollers or hot sticks.

Start by sectioning off the front and set it with three large rollers. Spray setting lotion on each section of hair before rolling. Brush the hair forwards, in front of the face, and roll each section under, starting with the middle roller.

Step 2

Set the back of the hair in rollers arranged in a horseshoe shape around the base of the head. To create a wave in the hair, roll the top row up and roll the rest of the rollers under. Roll the sides up and angle them slightly towards the back.

Brush each side up, style it into a roll, as described on page 79, and pin it on top of the head. Backcomb the fringe, roll it forward and pin it on the inside. Brush the back into shape, curling the ends under.

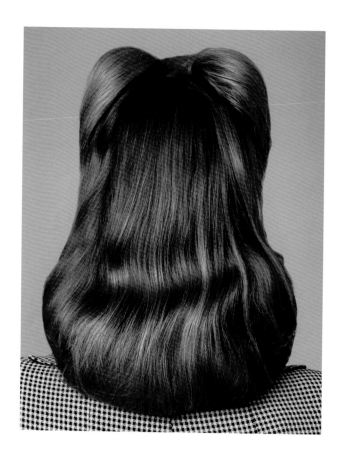

A set of long lashes gives
a simple, classic 1940s make-up
look an air of sophistication.

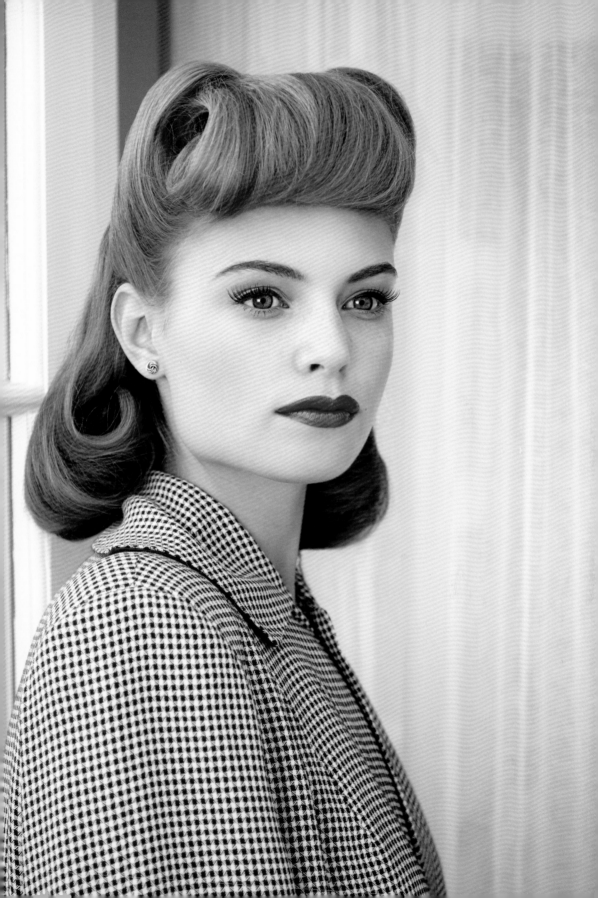

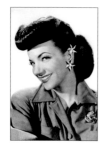

In a simple variation of the previous style, here, the hair at the back has been gathered up and secured in a clip at the nape of the neck. Our reference image shows Carmen Miranda sporting a particularly large rolled fringe. Hollywood stars tended to wear exaggerated, glamorous looks, whereas photographs of 'real' women of the time usually show more understated, simpler versions of the make-up and hairstyles presented on the silver screen – although there are, of course, always exceptions.

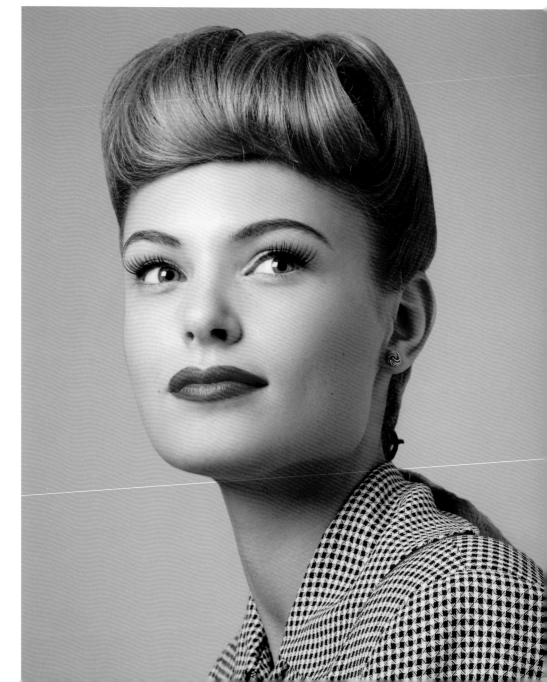

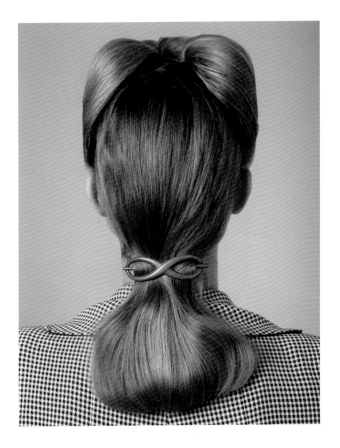

In the 1940s the emphasis was generally on the upper lashes, with only a faint application of mascara used on the bottom, if any at all.

Achieving the correct silhouettes
of the hairstyles of the era
is a crucial part of capturing
the look of the 1940s.

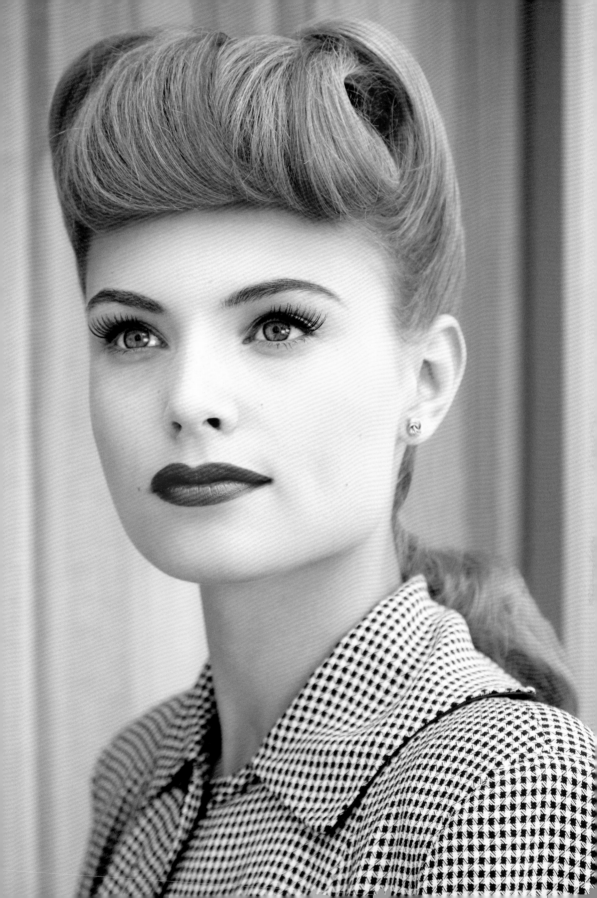

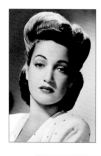

The Victory Roll, a look that was widely adopted in the 1940s, is purported to be named after an aerobatic manoeuvre carried out by fighter pilots in the Second World War as a sign of celebration. Women at the time achieved this style by simply wrapping a stocking around their head and then tucking the hair over the top of it, pinning it in place to create the desired shape. The look shown here features a Victory Roll at the back and a large wave at the front. The reference image is of Dorothy Lamour, who appeared in a series of popular comedies with Bob Hope and Bing Crosby.

THE

1940S

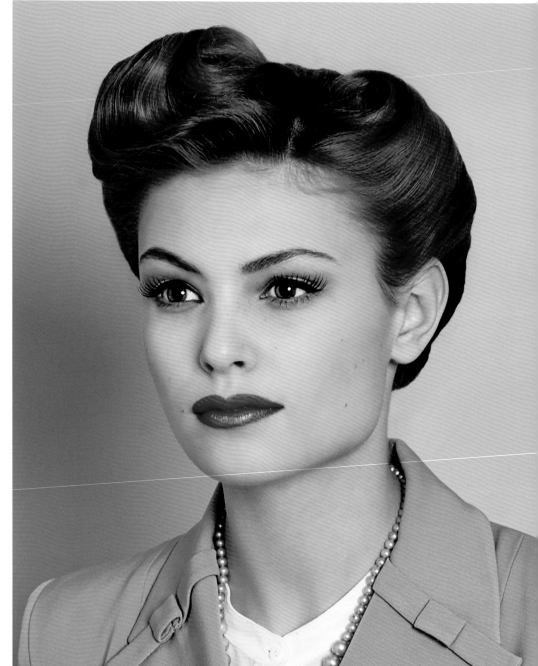

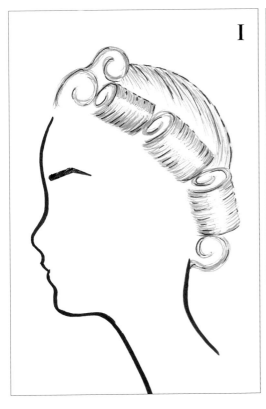

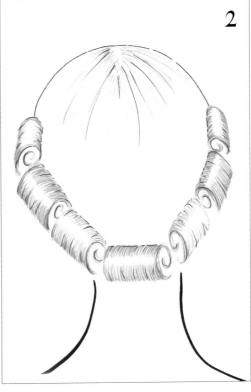

Step 1

Set the hair with medium heated rollers, as shown above. If the set is done accurately and neatly, the combing out will be easier.

Start with the front and side sections, rolling the hair away from the face, towards the parting, in the direction you want it to go. Spray each section with setting lotion. Now set the back of the hair in a horseshoe shape, creating a ring of rollers at the nape. The set should be exactly the same shape as the style when combed out.

Step 2

When the rollers have cooled, remove them and comb out the hair, beginning at the centre back. Put a little serum in your palm and stroke it through the hair as you comb. You may find it helpful to put a row of hair clips around the back of the head, about 2.5cm (1 in) up from

nape, so you can pin into them when creating the roll. If the hair is not very long, use padding, such as crepe wool or similar, to achieve the shape. Either roll up the hair, stuff with some padding and secure with a hair pin, or place the padding at the end of the section of hair and roll up towards the nape, then pin in place.

Comb out the sides, putting a little backcombing into the roots. Smooth the hair and roll round your finger in the direction of the roll at the back. Join up the rolls and secure with a hair grip.

Brush through the front, putting a little backcombing into the roots. Brush back and roll hair under at the same time, then push forward to make the wave. For a deeper wave, use marcel irons or waving clips.

Lou added a slide at the back to complete the look.

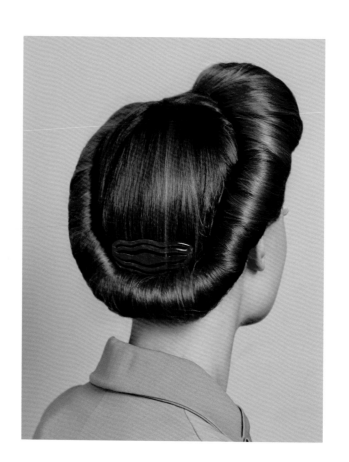

Padding was often used
to add volume to the
hairstyles of the 1940s.

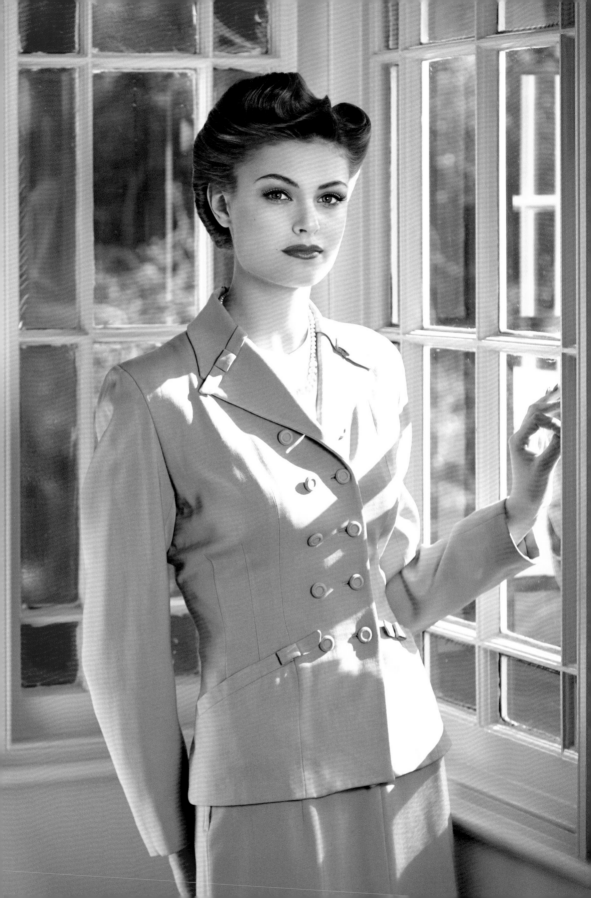

Some 1940s photographs show exaggeratedly overdrawn lips, but this requires a lot of maintenance. As long as you achieve the correct rounded lip shape, the look of the era is instantly recognizable.

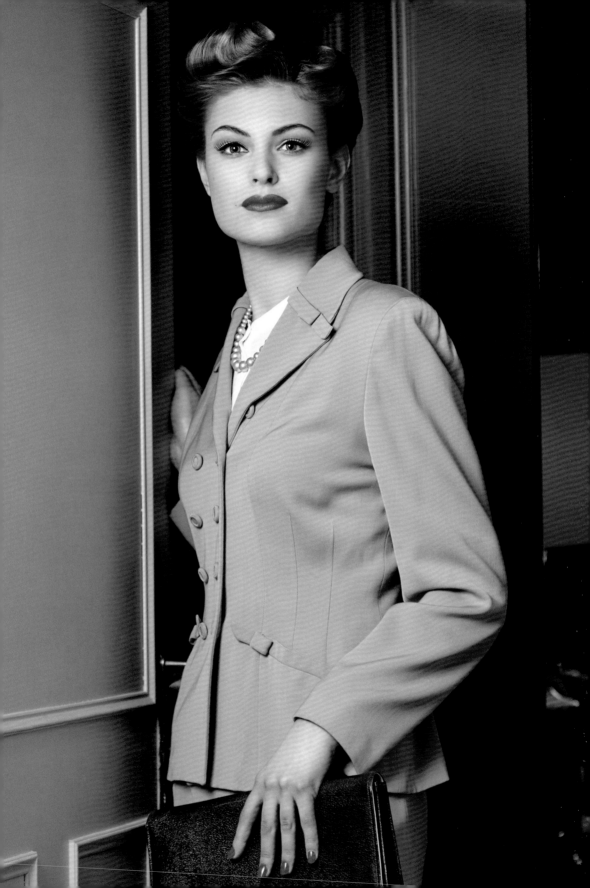

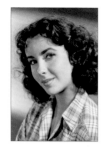

A simple look for a young girl. Our reference image here shows a youthful Elizabeth Taylor and, as a teenager in 1946, Princess Margaret also wore a similar style. Waves and curls were the height of fashion, and women and girls used a number of methods to achieve these looks at home.

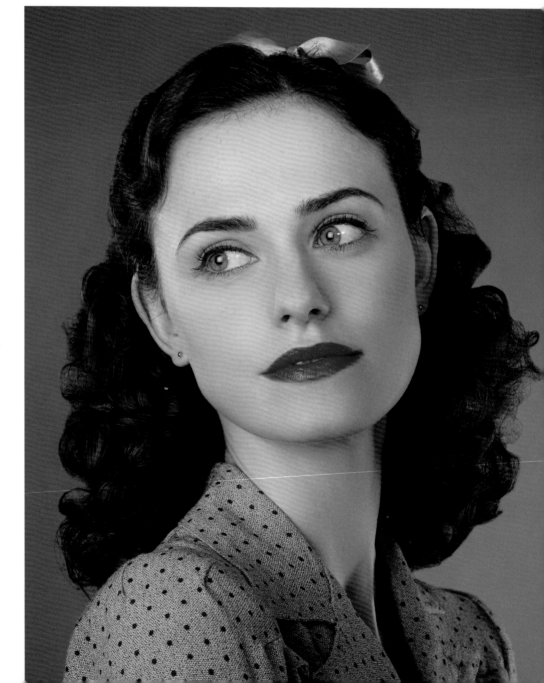

THE
—
1940S

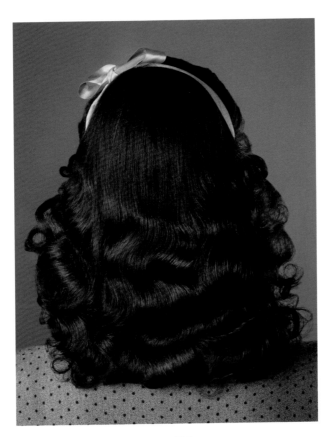

Make-up variation

Apply foundation, followed by
concealer (as needed) and
powder, as described in step 1 on
page 19 to create a flawless finish.

Keep the eyebrows neat but
natural, and define the eyes with
pencil eyeliner and a little mascara.

Add a touch of blusher for a
healthy glow, and finish off this
simple look with deep red
lipstick for a classic 1940s mouth.

Hair

This style was created with
heated rollers using the basic
1940s set shown on page 77.

Remove the cooled rollers and
brush the hair through to create
natural waves. Style it with a
ribbon tied into a bow.

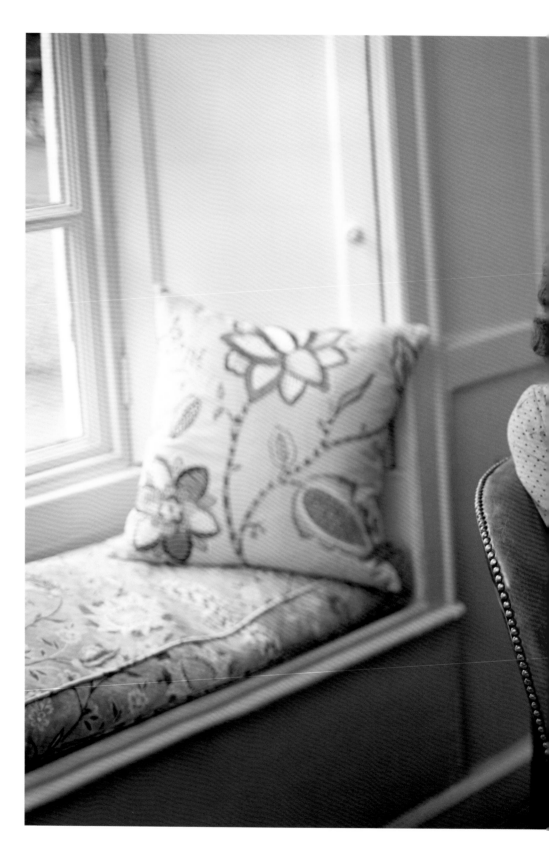

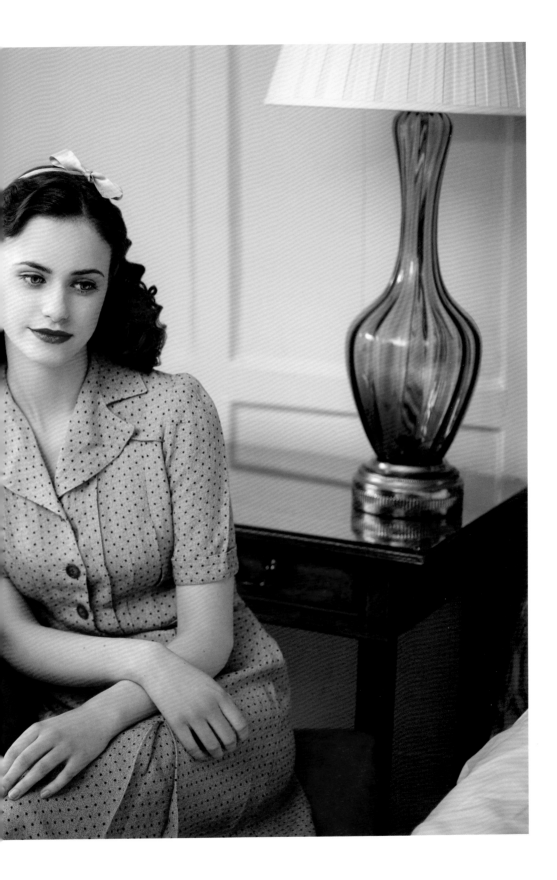

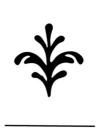

The 1950s

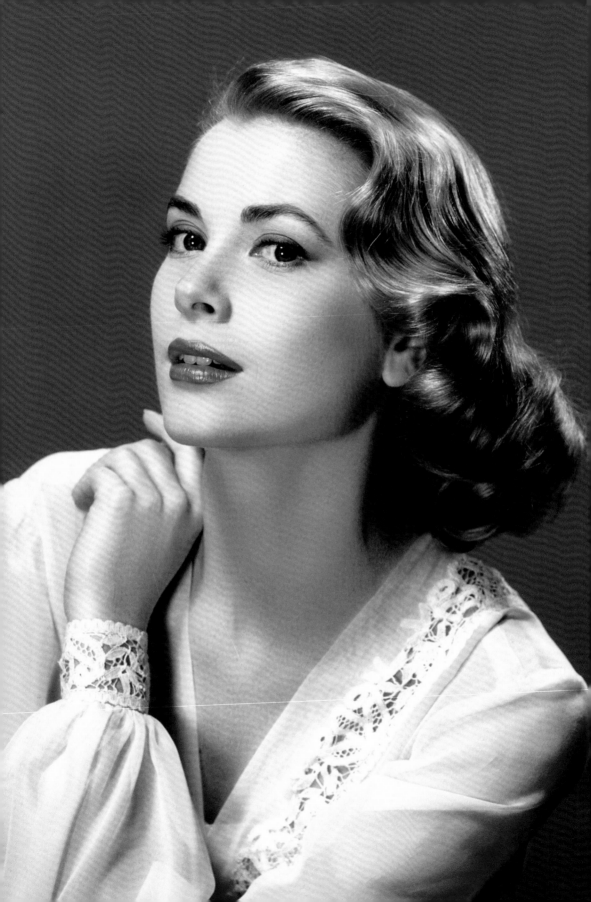

The 1950s

AFTER THE AUSTERITY OF THE 1940S, THE WORLD WELCOMED THE 1950S WITH OPTIMISM. MANY OF THE MAKE-UP AND HAIR TRENDS OF THE ERA ARE AS RELEVANT TODAY AS WHEN THEY FIRST EMERGED AND HAVE REMAINED POPULAR EVER SINCE.

The rationing of some products continued into the early 1950s in the UK, but in the USA it ended not long after the Second World War. Production boomed again and women had a greater choice of cosmetics.

MAKE-UP

In the 1950s, make-up looks were simple, elegant and strong. Advertisements and even popular songs encouraged women to make the best of themselves and make-up was widely used. Women matched their nail varnish to their lipstick, in colours such as red, coral and pink. They wore eyeshadow in blue, green, soft brown and lilac, with eyeliner that was flicked at the ends.

The doe-eyed look made an impact early in the decade, heralding a new look for women. It was famously featured on the beautiful model Jean Patchett, as photographed by Erwin Blumenfeld for the cover of *Vogue* in 1950. Patchett, Suzy Parker, Lisa Fonssagrives and Dovima were among the first supermodels, and their ice-cool, aloof style reigned supreme until it was swept aside by a new breed of models in the 1960s.

The archetypal Hollywood blonde Marilyn Monroe was a massive box-office draw and her look spawned an array of copycats, from Jayne Mansfield to Diana Dors. Brunettes Elizabeth Taylor and Audrey Hepburn were much admired by men and women alike, as was the elegant beauty Grace Kelly. While Hollywood stars continued to set trends, the growing ownership of TV sets meant that a much larger audience was influenced by the women they saw on the small screen. The

coronation of Queen Elizabeth II in 1953 was the perfect reason for many British households to purchase their first TV set.

In the world of beauty products, Helena Rubinstein and Elizabeth Arden – still competing with each other – brought out luxury cosmetics and skin preparations.

The 1950s also saw the birth of the 'teenager' – the first time that young people were recognized as a separate group within society. Cosmetics companies and advertisers were quick to capitalize on their spending power by creating looks and products aimed at teens. The advent of rock and roll created yet another creative source of inspiration.

HAIR

The 1950s saw a variety of hair lengths and styles, ranging from pageboys, poodle cuts, bubble cuts, ponytails and elegant French pleats to the short 'Italian Boy' cut. Originating in Italy in the early 1950s, this style was soon widely adopted. Italian film stars such as Gina Lollobrigida wore this chic, short, softly curled look, tapered in at the neck, and variations soon appeared. The short, cropped version Audrey Hepburn wore in the 1953 film *Roman Holiday* cemented the popularity of the look.

Women loved to colour their hair, and new products made it easier for them to do so themselves at home. It was customary for women to wear hats, especially in the early 1950s, and so the hairstyles of the day were suitably compact to accommodate this. Towards the end of the decade hairstyles became softer and had more volume.

Opposite: Grace Kelly, 1955

After years of wartime restrictions, more cosmetics were available in the 1950s. New formulas made products easier to use and packaging became increasingly sophisticated. Max Factor continued to develop innovative products, such as the first complete foundation, called Creme Puff, which was launched in 1953. It was followed in 1954 by Erace, the first concealer stick. The company's Pan-Cake foundation continued to be very popular.

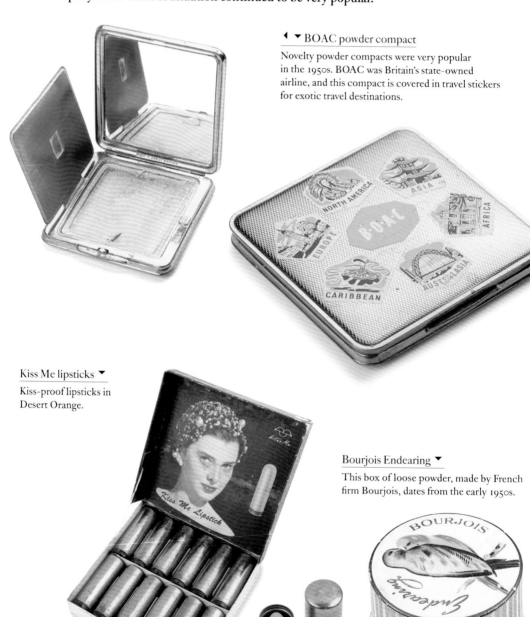

◀ ▼ BOAC powder compact
Novelty powder compacts were very popular in the 1950s. BOAC was Britain's state-owned airline, and this compact is covered in travel stickers for exotic travel destinations.

Kiss Me lipsticks ▼
Kiss-proof lipsticks in Desert Orange.

Bourjois Endearing ▼
This box of loose powder, made by French firm Bourjois, dates from the early 1950s.

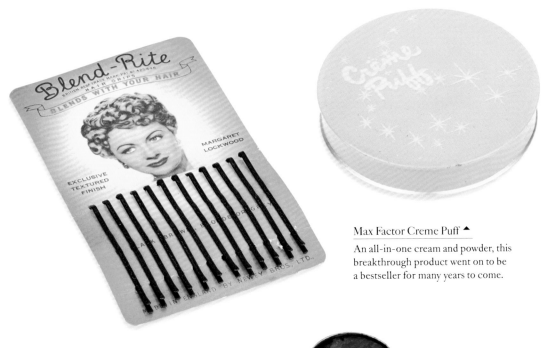

Max Factor Creme Puff ▲

An all-in-one cream and powder, this breakthrough product went on to be a bestseller for many years to come.

Blend-Rite hairgrips ▲

Even hairgrips (bobby pins) were endorsed by celebrities: this packaging features the British actress Margaret Lockwood.

Mirrored lip compact ▲

The handle of this lip mirror from the early 1950s contains a lip brush, while the centre of the compact rotates to reveal the lip colour.

Helena Rubinstein false lashes ▶

False eyelashes were first available in the early 20th century, but their use became more widespread in the 1920s and 1930s largely due to the influence of Hollywood. They grew in popularity again in the late 1950, before the 1960s saw them become an essential part of a woman's make-up.

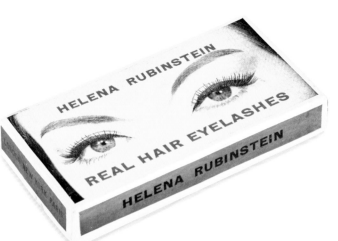

As the restrictions imposed during the war years began to be lifted, the 1950s saw a wider range of make-up colours become available. Lipstick was a mainstay of the era's classic looks, and colours ranged from a Marilyn-Monroe-esque red to vibrant pinks and oranges. The doe-eyed look introduced at the start of the decade featured more emphasis on the eyes, which were lined top and bottom and flicked at the outer corners. Women adapted this look, credited as coming from France, in various ways.

The glamorous style of the 1950s is associated with red-carpet looks the world over.

LIPSTICK

Well-known colours of the 1950s include Revlon's Fire and Ice – a 'lush and passionate scarlet', in the words of the advertising poster – as well as Elizabeth Arden's Arden Pink and Revlon's Love that Pink.

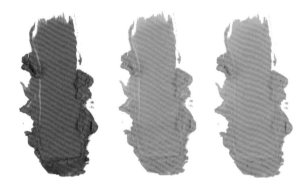

EYESHADOW

Green, blue and brown were all popular colours for eyeshadow. The eyes were lined with pencils or cake liners.

BLUSHER

Minimal blusher was used for many looks of the era – just a touch of coral, pink or rose.

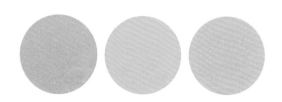

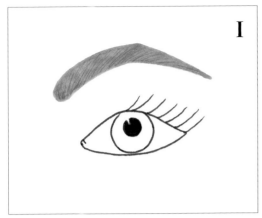

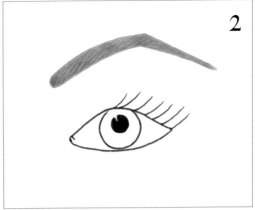

Brows Look 1

Strong, angled brows were worn throughout the 1950s. Although at some points a softer angle was adopted, brows were still kept more prominent in this decade than in the 1940s.

Brows Look 2

Dark, sharply angled brows accompanied the doe-eyed look of the early 1950s. Sometimes a high arch was preferred.

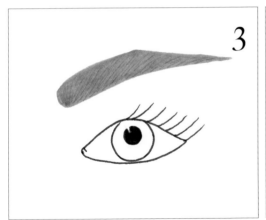

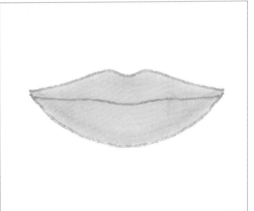

Brows Look 3

Audrey Hepburn's overdrawn brows angled upwards and out – possibly originating from the Mandarin look that saw a more extreme, straighter version of this shape.

Lips

The lips were not overdrawn, as they had been in the 1940s, but were still a main feature, with full, luscious lips being a focal point of the popular looks of the decade.

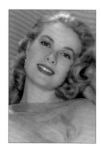

This is a classic 1950s look, as seen in our reference picture of Grace Kelly. Known for her style and ice-cool elegance, she was a Hollywood princess before becoming a real one in Monaco when she married Prince Ranier III in 1956. This waved pageboy was a popular hairstyle and was seen on shorter hair, too. The make-up shown here is a simple 1950s style (see Look 5, pages 153–4). Some women used cake liner to define their eyes, while others used pencil. For a more glamorous Hollywood look, false lashes can be used, but leave them off for a simpler style.

THE

1950S

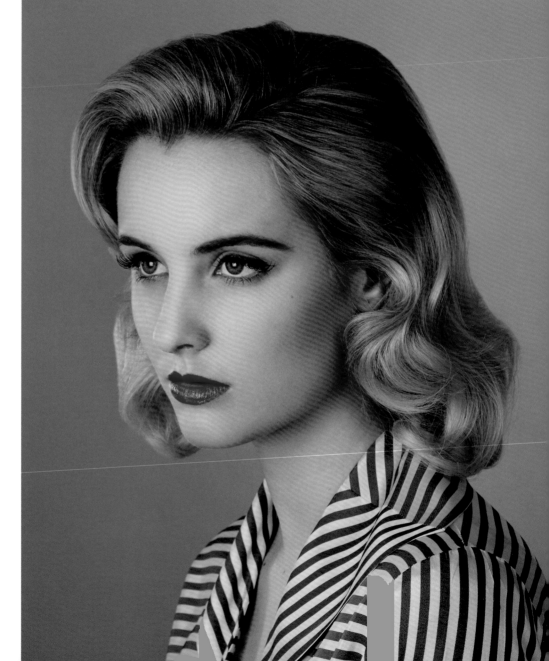

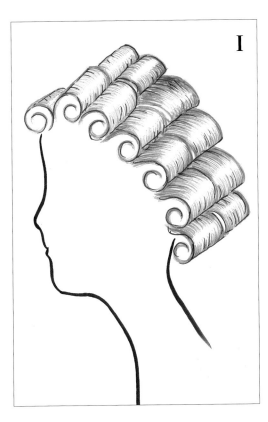

Step 1

Although this look is simple to style, the correct set is essential in order to achieve the desired effect.

Set the hair on medium-sized heated rollers in the direction shown above. Remove the rollers when they have cooled.

To dress the hair, just brush it through, sweep the front section over to one side and push the waves away from the face and into place. You can backcomb the front section slightly to give a little more volume and height.

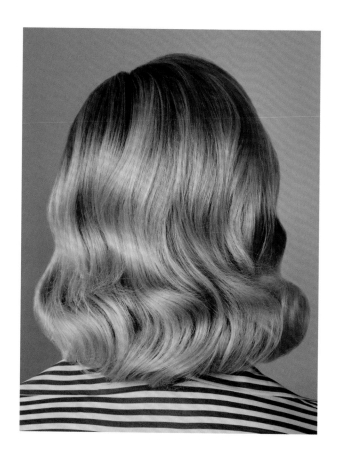

This simple and elegant
waved pageboy style is
flattering to shorter cuts as
well as mid-length hair.

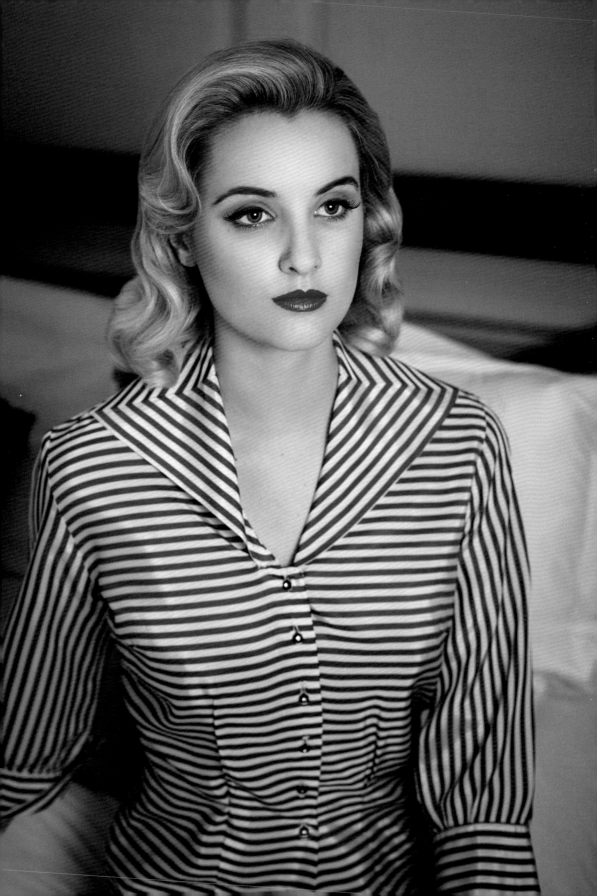

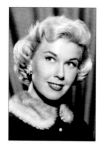

Our inspirations for this hairstyle were the girl-next-door looks that became so popular in the mid-1950s, as many women began to aspire to a more effortless natural glamour. Our reference image shows the actress Doris Day, who epitomizes an easier-to-attain glamour than some of the more aloof, untouchable stars of the previous decades. As the decade advanced and the wearing of hats gradually became less popular, the flatter styles that had prevailed in the early part of the decade started to become more bouffant. The make-up shown here is a variation on Look 5 (see pages 153–4).

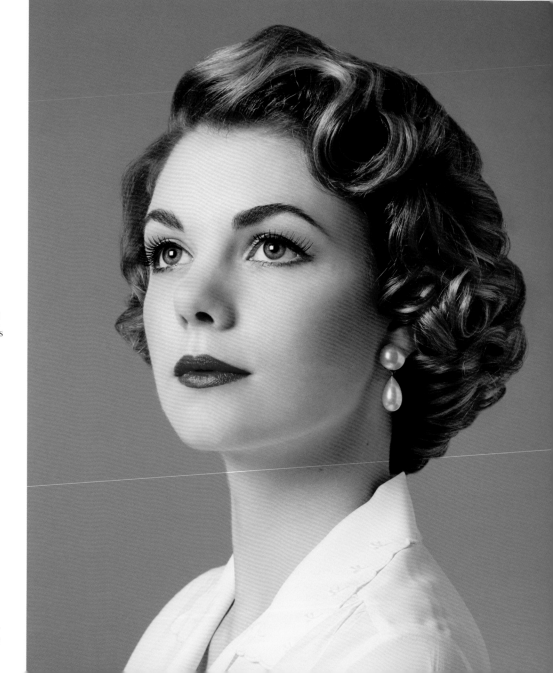

THE

1950S

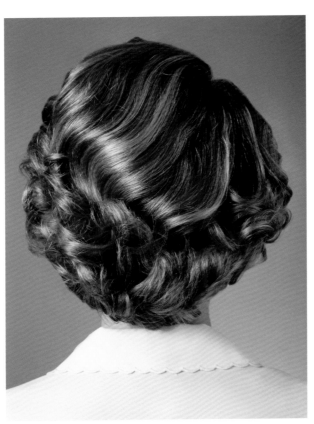

Make-up variation

Arch the brows using an angled
brow brush and matte eyeshadow.
Emphasize the eyelid with a little
natural shadow. Apply cake liner in
very dark brown along the upper
lash line, and then use a dark brown
pencil liner under the eye at the
outer corner. Many women adopted
this more understated approach to
the doe-eyed look, rather than some
of the more extreme versions of
under-eye shading. Apply dark
brown mascara, and add lashes for a
more glamorous look.

Accentuate the cheeks with a
minimal touch of blusher, and
complete the look with full, red lips.

Hair

The hair is a soft, curled and natural
version of the set on page 155. This
was a much-worn style that could be
clipped up at the side as a variation.

To style, just remove the cooled
rollers and brush the hair into shape.
If need be, redefine the curls by
twisting them around your finger
and arranging them place.

This is a stand-out style
from the 1950s – both make-up
and hair look as fresh today
as they did then.

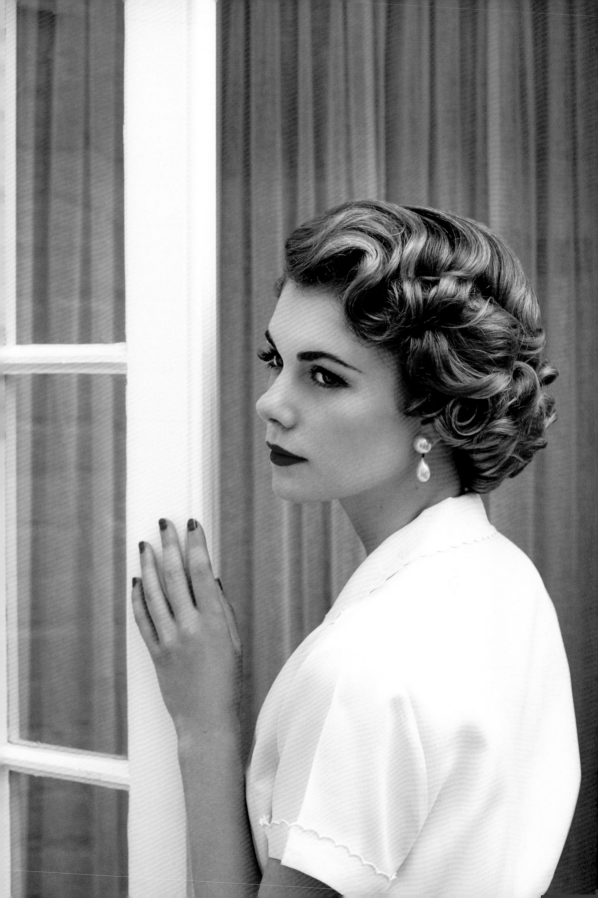

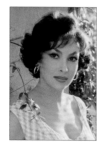

European actresses coming into Hollywood in the 1950s, such as Gina Lollobrigida (pictured here) and Sophia Loren, both from Italy, introduced a new dimension to the film industry and went on to influence the public. The make-up is an elegant variation of the previous look, with lilac eyeshadow and a pink-red lip. The hair has movement and the soft curls frame the face.

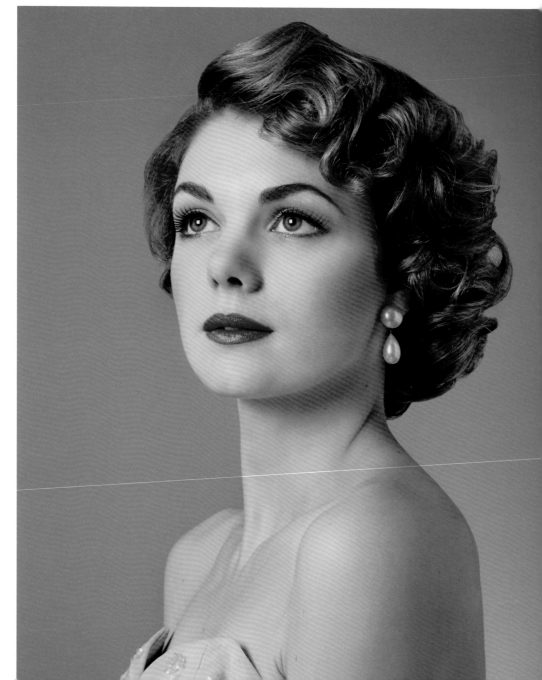

THE
1950S

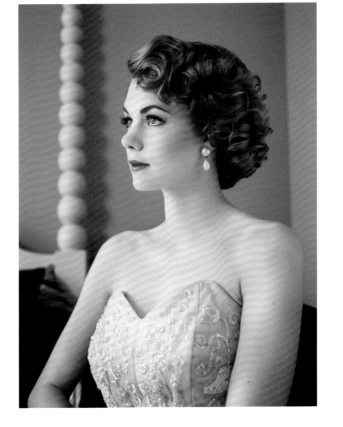

This flattering look was
seen at many proms,
dances and debutante
balls in the 1950s.

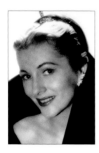

This classic French pleat is an elegant look still worn today. This more dramatic look was seen on many fashion models of the 1950s. I shaded the eyes in brown matte shadow and applied black cake liner and flicked this upwards and outwards at the eye corners. Minimal blusher and a bright red lipstick complete the look. Our reference image is of Joan Fontaine, who first rose to fame in the film adaptation of Daphne du Maurier's *Rebecca*, directed by Alfred Hitchcock in 1940, and went on to star in numerous melodramas.

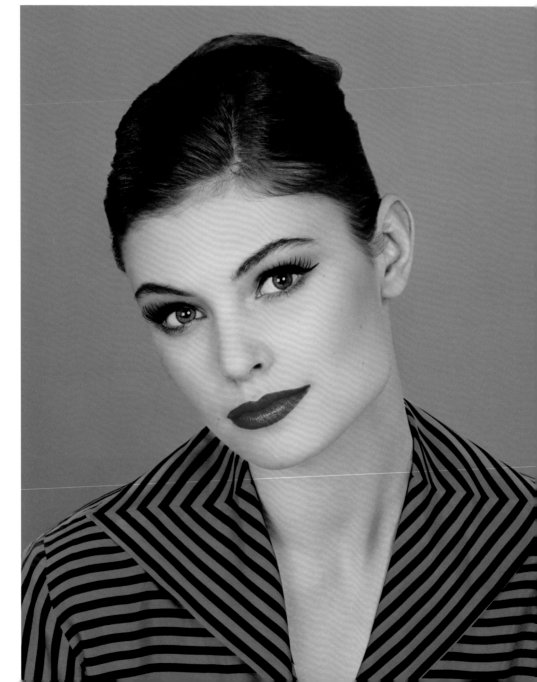

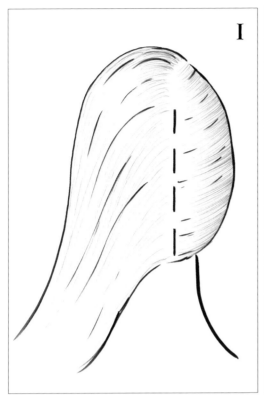

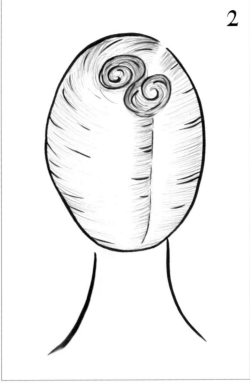

Step 1

Brush the right side of the hair over to the left and insert hairgrips (bobby pins) in a straight line up the centre back of the head.

Step 2

Take the left side of the hair and fold in to the right, twisting and lifting to make the pleat.

Angle the hair up and insert grips into the fold to secure it, then style the ends as desired.

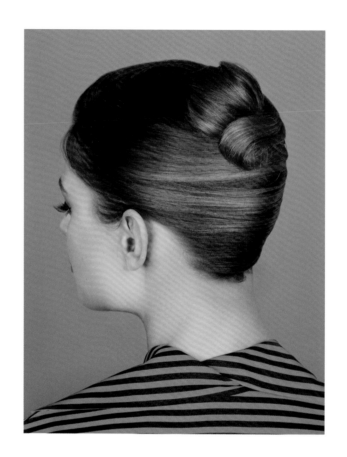

This sleek, simple version
of a classic French pleat is
ideal for wearing under a hat
(see page 150).

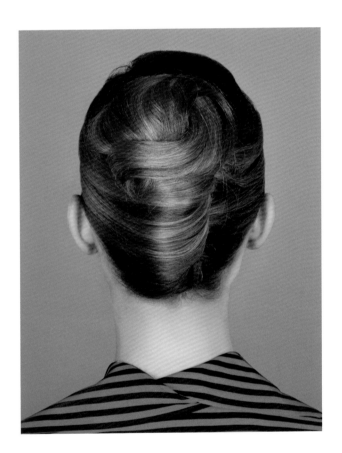

This hairstyle lends itself particularly well to being worn with adornments, clips and slides for any formal occasion.

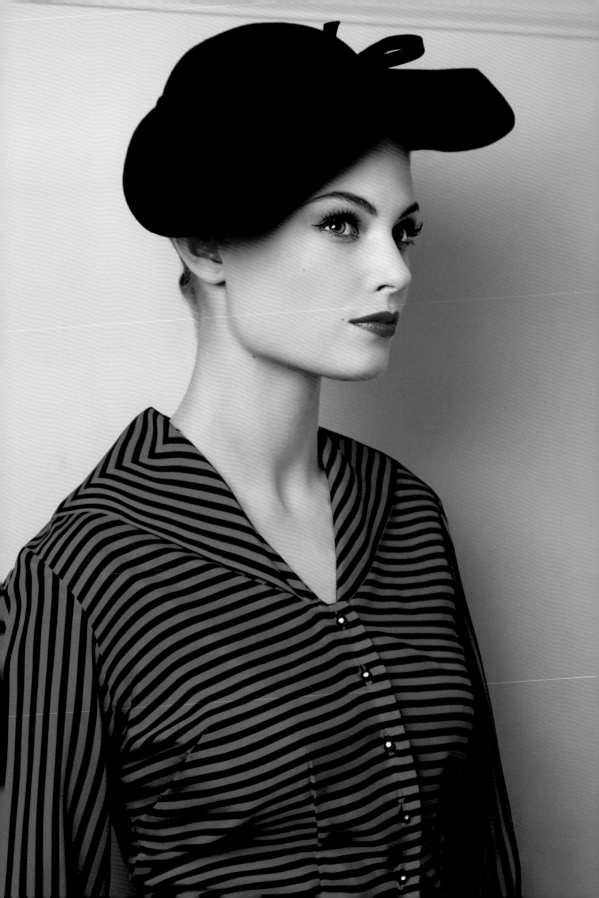

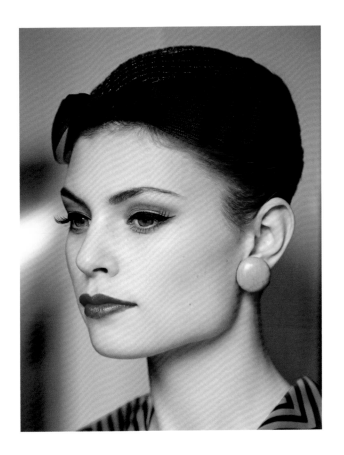

This look works well on larger eyelids – if you have smaller lids, use a thinner line.

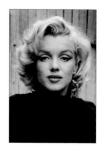

Our reference for this look is Marilyn Monroe, probably the most famous blonde bombshell of all time. The iconic star often wore hairstyles that were more 'done' than this, including a shorter version of the curled-under waved pageboy shown on page 136. This photograph shows her with a relatively relaxed style of both hair and make-up, which nevertheless exudes glamour and remains many people's definitive image of the 1950s.

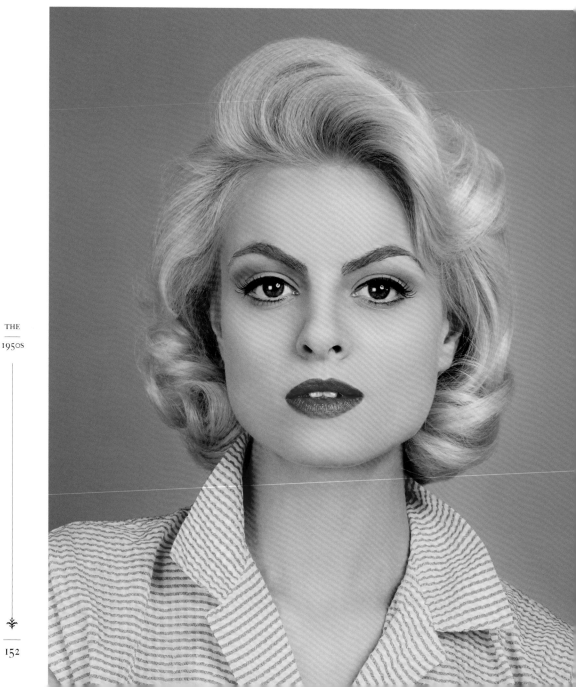

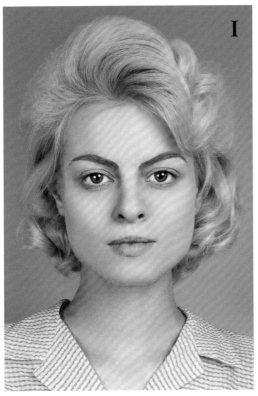

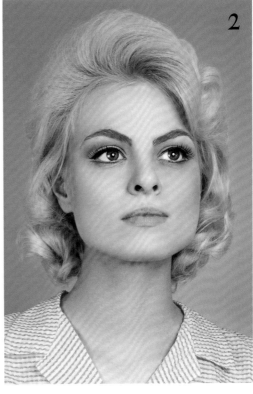

Step 1

Foundation: At the time Pan-Cake and Pan-Stik were among the most popular foundations and widely promoted by Hollywood celebrities.

Apply foundation, followed by concealer and powder, as described in step 1 on page 19.

Brows: Apply matte shadow or brow powder to the brows with a firm, angled brow brush. Keep the angled edge of the brush sharp by wetting it.

Create the brow arch, if need be, by applying more colour to the top of the brow where you want the arch to be. Elongate the brows with the brow colour, as necessary.

Check that the brows don't look too drawn on and brush them through for a softer look.

Step 2

Eyeshadow: Apply a pale matte base shadow all over the lid and up to the eyebrow. Shade the socket and brow bone with a mid-toned peachy brown shadow.

Apply black cake liner to the top lash line, flicking it out and up slightly. Draw a soft line under the eye with a brown pencil and extend this out, parallel with the top line. Using a white pencil, draw a faint line between these two lines – the cake liner and the under-eye line – at the outer corner of the eye. Distinctive to Marilyn's eye make-up, this is based on theatrical make-up. On the whole, other make-up looks of the 1950s did not include this white line.

Lashes: Apply black mascara to the top and bottom lashes. Add false lashes to the top lids and go over the cake liner afterwards to conceal where the lashes are attached.

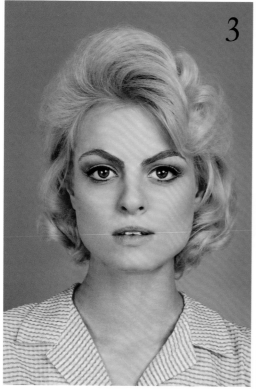

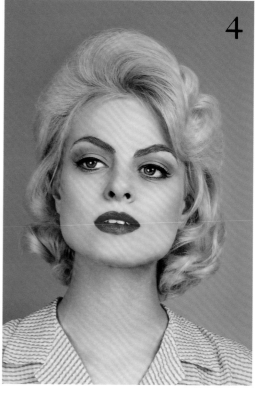

Step 3

Blusher: Using a blusher brush, blend a soft peach-toned powder blusher on to the cheekbones. This mirrors the peach tone I used on the brow bone and lifts the eye.

Step 4

Lipstick: Choose a vibrant red lip colour and matching lip pencil.

Outline the lips with the pencil and then use a lip brush to fill in the shape with the bright red lip colour.

In the 1950s the lips were not overdrawn as they were in the previous decade, but make sure that the whole lip area is filled in to give a full shape. It helps to open the mouth so you can get right to the corners of the lips with the lipstick – and of course, use a good brush.

Classic Marilyn Monroe – arguably the most famous make-up and hair look of the 20th century.

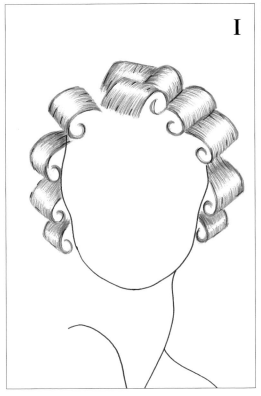

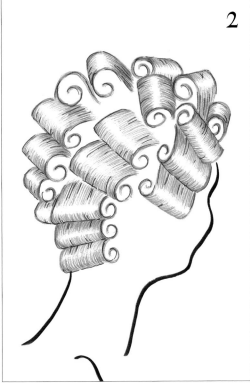

Step 1

Set the hair, as shown above, on large heated rollers. Start with the front and side sections of hair, making sure the rollers are angled in the direction you want the hair to go when you style it. Notice how the front roller is set back here to create the front lift in the final style.

Step 2

Set the back of the hair in the same way, remembering that if the set is correct, the resulting curls will naturally fall into the right place.

When the rollers have cooled, remove them and brush the hair loosely into style.

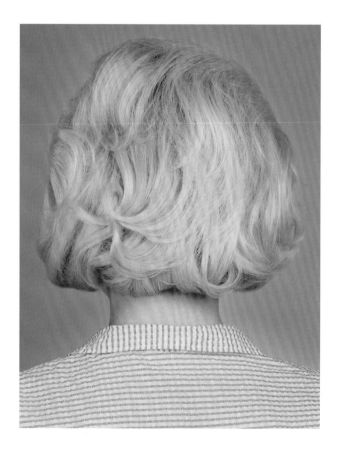

A real Hollywood style that
looks as good today as it did
in the 1950s. This look was
copied the world over and
is still instantly recognized
as belonging to this era.

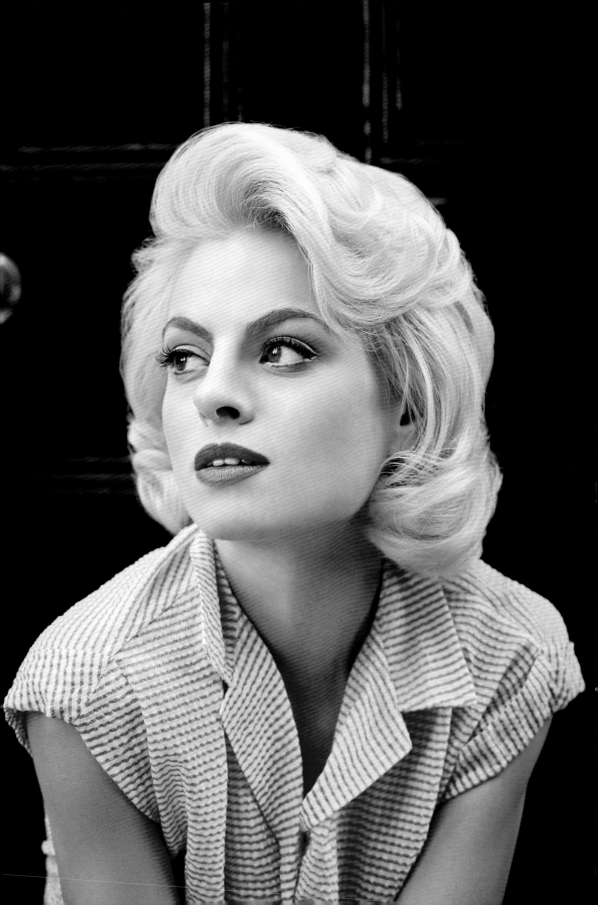

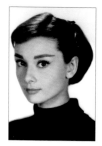

The late 1950s saw teenagers identified as a distinct group for the first time, and this provided many opportunities for cosmetics and hair companies to create products aimed at a younger market. The popular ponytail is an ultra-simple style that looks youthful and fun. Worn by music stars and film stars alike, the ponytail was often set off by a short fringe. Our reference photograph here shows the beautiful Audrey Hepburn.

THE
1950S

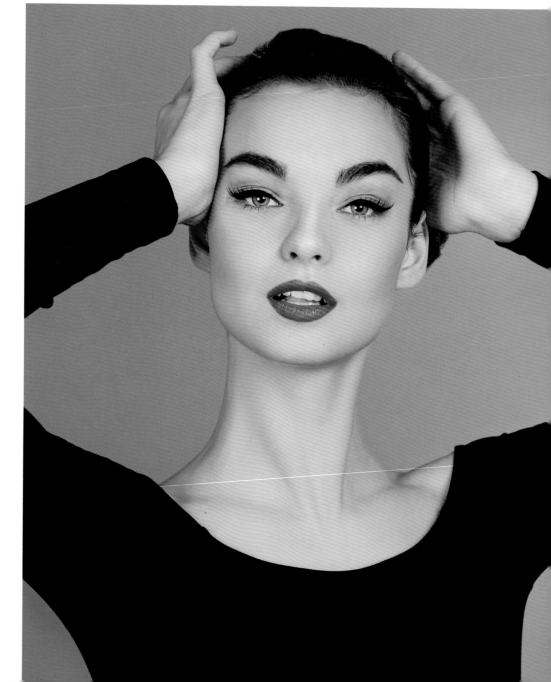

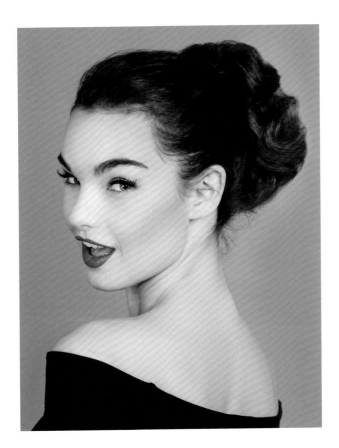

Make-up variation

Angle and shape the eyebrows,
as shown in Look 3 on page 135.

Apply eyeliner on the top lash
lines only and angle it upwards.

Use a little tan/brown shadow to
shade the top lids only.

Keep the blusher to a minimum
and add full red lips for a really
simple 1950s look.

Hair

Pull the hair into a high pony tail,
secure with a hairband and curl
with two or three heated rollers.

When you have removed the
cooled rollers, brush out the hair
and add a ribbon if you wish.

In the 1950s, longer hair could be worn loose or in a high ponytail, often tied with a ribbon – a look that was popular with teenagers.

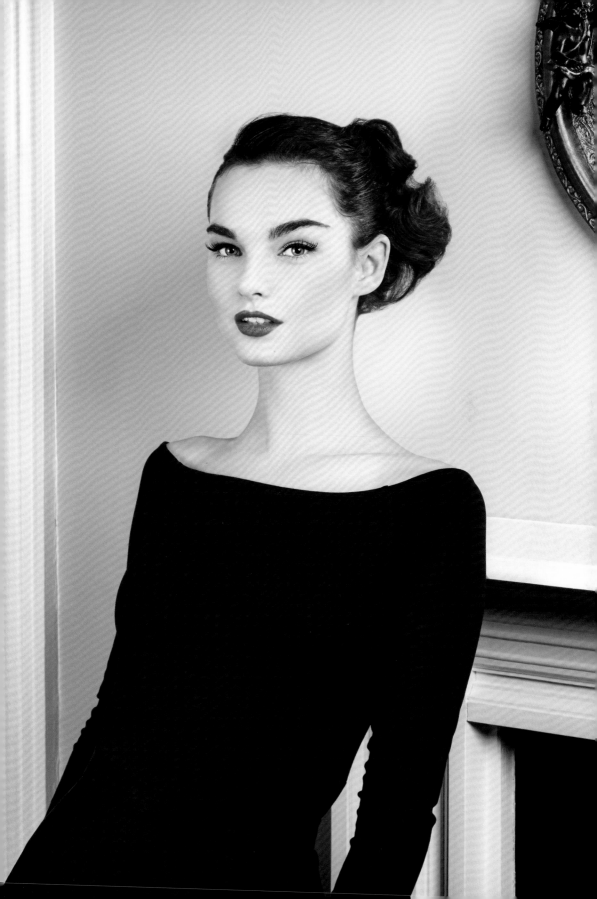

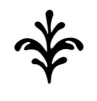

The 1960s

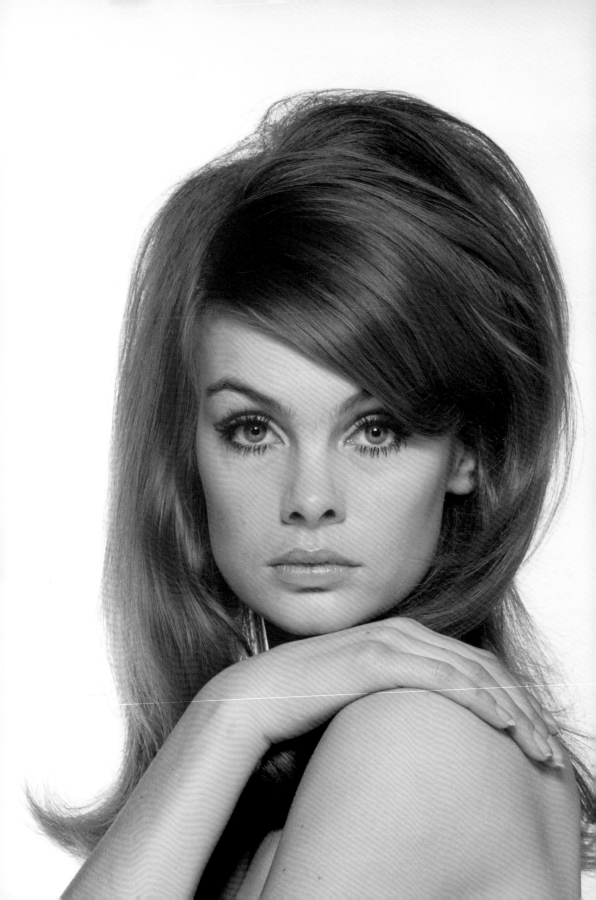

The 1960s

MY PASSION FOR MAKE-UP STARTED AS A CHILD IN THE LATE 1960S. I WOULD WATCH, FASCINATED, AS MY COUSIN MADE UP HER EYES: THE DEFINITE SOCKET LINE, FLICKED LINER, CAREFULLY PAINTED-IN LASHES ON THE BOTTOM LID, ALL FINISHED OFF WITH TWO PAIRS OF LASHES ON THE TOP AND ONE ON THE BOTTOM. I WAS HOOKED!

In the 1950s, girls copied their mothers' hair and make-up, but by the end of the decade the influence of pop music, as well as changing social attitudes, led to a new freedom in the way young people expressed themselves through their make-up, hair and clothes.

MAKE-UP

The Beatles took the world by storm, models Jean Shrimpton and Twiggy made their mark, and designer Mary Quant created fun fashions that influenced make-up as London became a fashion hub. The older generation began copying the style leaders – the young.

The flicked eye lines and pastel blue or green shadows of the late 1950s carried over into the early 1960s, but new looks soon emerged. One of the decade's biggest trends was inspired by Elizabeth Taylor's appearance in the 1963 film *Cleopatra*. Her make-up design was a 1960s take on ancient Egypt, and make-up companies were quick to market products to achieve the look.

Towards the mid-1960s, the defined eye sockets and drawn-on lashes made popular by Twiggy were interpreted by women at home – with mixed results. They applied dramatic eye lines with cake or pencil eyeliner, and often layered cake mascara to give a thick-lash effect. Some women plucked their brows into non-existence, while others left them more natural. False lashes were worn in the day and evening, while lips were pale or natural to keep the emphasis on the eyes.

Later a more bohemian influence came into play, with some girls opting for a completely natural look. The hippy Woodstock spirit inspired a trend for face and body painting, with model Verushka being a fan.

The Biba look, born when the eponymous London store opened in the mid-1960s, was all about dark plum, bottle-green and navy blue shadows and coordinating blusher and lipstick. Different from the other 1960s styles, it was reminiscent of 1920s vamps.

My favourite look was that of singer Julie Driscoll. Like a psychedelic fairy, she sported a short pixie crop and eye make-up that often featured little stars, lips blanked out with concealer and shading under her cheeks.

HAIR

Various hairstyles were popular at the time, and a feature many of them had in common was height at the crown. Whether it was for a beehive or a bouffant flick-up, backcombing played a big part in 1960s hairstyling. Hairpieces, added to create an instant hairstyle or extra volume, were also popular.

Throughout the decade hairstylist Vidal Sassoon created his innovative signature angled bobs for the likes of Mary Quant, model Grace Coddington and actresses Mia Farrow and Nancy Kwan. Inspired by 1920s bobs, his geometric but natural shapes cut down on the need for hairspray and accentuated the hair's natural shine.

Later in the decade, longer, hippy-influenced styles started to emerge. Women of colour who had straightened their hair in the 1940s and 1950s began leaving it natural and teasing their curls into Afros – a look that reached its peak in the 1970s.

Opposite: Jean Shrimpton, c.1965

The cultural revolution of the 1960s saw innovative make-up formulations produced, boundaries being pushed and the youthful Swinging London scene influencing looks the world over. Fashion designer Mary Quant launched her make-up up range in 1966; other popular cosmetics brands of the time include Max Factor, Yardley, Revlon, Coty, Elizabeth Arden and Helena Rubinstein.

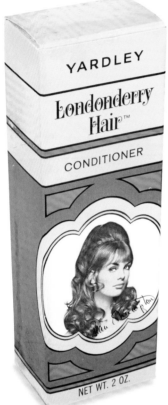

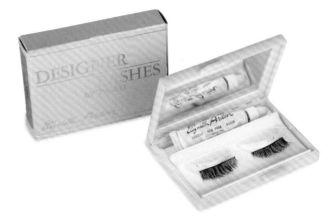

◀ Yardley hair conditioner

Model Jean Shrimpton is featured on the packaging of this conditioner. Jean modelled for Yardley during the 1960s, advertising the company's London Look collection.

▲ Elizabeth Arden lashes

These lashes were designed for Elizabeth Arden by the company's Italian make-up artist Pablo. Increasingly, cosmetics companies worked with make-up artists to design their seasonal looks.

▼ Pond's make-up set

This Angel Face make-up set produced by Pond's dates from the early 1960s.

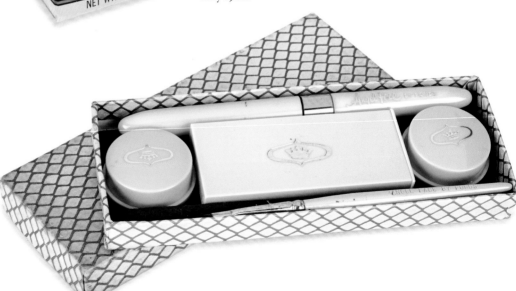

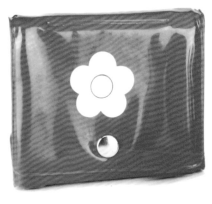

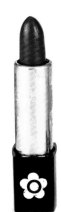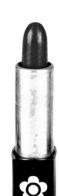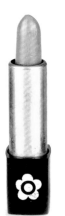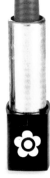

Mary Quant make-up ▲

The cool, mod design of Mary Quant's
make-up packaging caught the imagination
of the younger end of the market.

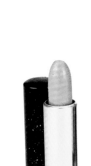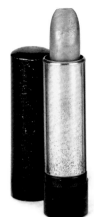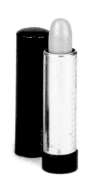

▼ Baby Doll lipstick

The Baby Doll range was sold in
Woolworths stores in Britain in the
late 1960s. Pinky Brown is a typically
pale 1960s colour.

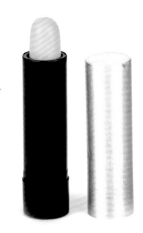

Lipstick colours ▲

The 1960s saw lip colours produced in a new spectrum
of shades, such as gold, silver and white, as well as
frosted lilacs and blues.

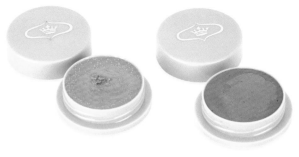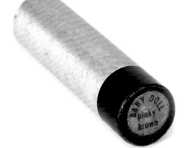

Pond's eyeshadows ▲

The Angel Face line included cream eyeshadows.

The general trend was to emphasize the eyes, rather than the mouth or cheeks. As the middle of the decade approached, this trend reached a peak, with very pale lips and minimal blusher paired with coloured eyes, often contrasting shades applied in sharp, unblended lines. The early 1960s saw shading and highlighting (now better known as contouring) become popular. Women used tan shaders and frosted highlighters to attempt to change the shape of their faces, sometimes resulting in an unfortunate streaky-looking effect.

> Layering two or even three pairs of false eyelashes on the top lid was not uncommon.

LIPSTICK

As is always the case, colours from the late 1950s were still being used in the early 1960s. Lip colours were available in numerous shades and textures through the decade, with pale shades being particularly fashionable.

EYE MAKE-UP

Shadows in pastel shades were popular, as were dark shadows or pencils used to define socket lines. Liquid and cake liner was available in many shades, including a shiny white version by Max Factor. Lashes came in every shape and size imaginable, including strips that could be cut to the required length. Bottom lashes were also popular. Some girls painted on eyelashes – a look made famous by Twiggy – with varying degrees of success. The most accurate results were achieved with a fine liner brush, while using an eye pencil resulted in thick, stubby-looking drawn-on lashes.

BLUSHER

Cheek colour was often minimal, in pale pink or peach tones, with tan popular for shading under the cheekbones. In the late 1960s blushing gels and stick blusher/bronzers heralded a more sun-kissed trend. Revlon Face Gleamers launched in 1967 and were a huge success.

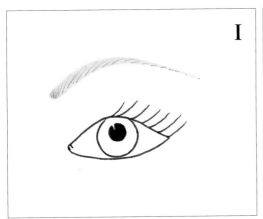

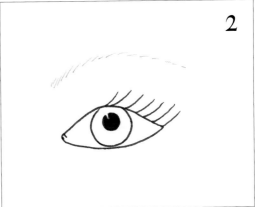

Brows Look 1

At the beginning of the decade, brows were fuller, with a thinner shape becoming popular in the middle years. The hippy trend at the end of the decade saw eyebrows return to a more natural shape.

Brows Look 2

Towards the middle of the 1960s, the fashionable brow was a very fine, almost non-existent line.

The trend for placing all the emphasis on the eye make-up meant that brows were made increasingly invisible – by plucking, bleaching or in some cases even covering them up with foundation.

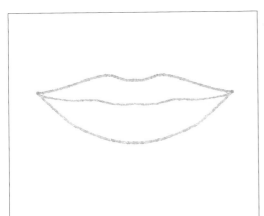

Lips

In the very early 1960s, the pinks and deep corals that were fashionable in the late 1950s were still popular.

As the decade wore on, the most fashionable lips were pale, and in some cases even completely concealed with foundation.

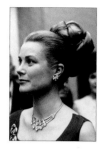

The make-up and hair of the 1960s are among the most easily recognizable styles of the 20th century, and still influence fashion today. This look would have been worn for a cocktail party or evening occasion. Our reference image shows Princess Grace of Monaco (formerly known as Grace Kelly) wearing a similar look in the 1960s. Today, a version of this look would be ideal for proms and parties or even weddings.

THE
1960S

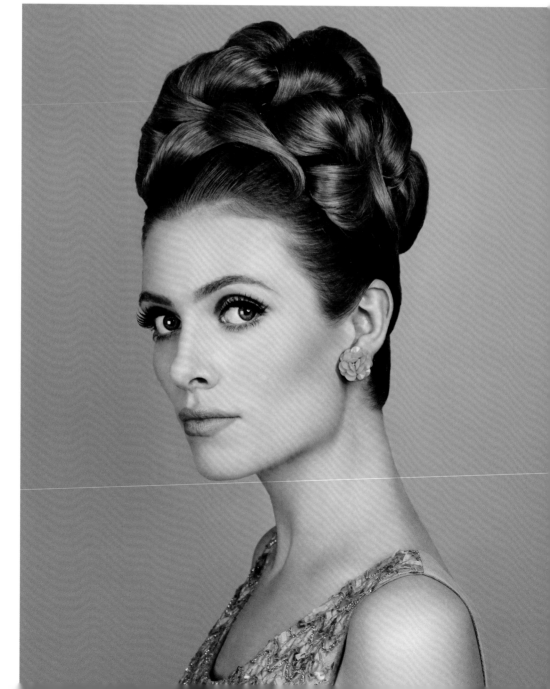

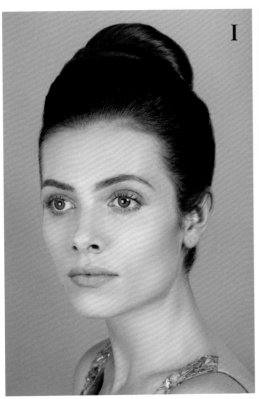

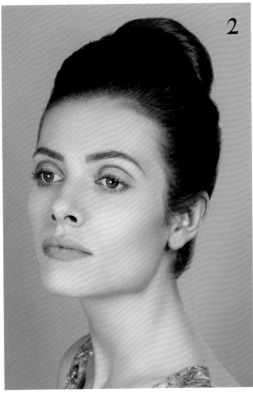

Step 1

Foundation: Apply foundation, followed by concealer and powder, as described in step 1 on page 19.

Brows: I kept the eyebrows natural for this look. If necessary, fill in any gaps and neaten the shape using an angled brow brush and matte brow powder or an eyeshadow the same colour as the brow.

Step 2

Eyeshadow: Apply a matte base shadow in a light cream colour over the entire eyelid and up to the brow.

Using a small pencil socket brush, apply brown eyeshadow to the socket line in a definite line. Finish the line at the outer corner of the eye, fading it to a point at the end.

It is important to get this socket line in exactly the right position, as otherwise it can make the eye appear to droop. If you are unsure, blend the upper edge of the sharp line slightly upwards, without altering its shape, so the colour fades out softly above the line, as in Look 2 on page 178.

Using a fine eyeliner brush, apply black cake liner to the upper lash line and flick it out very slightly at the outer corner of the eye.

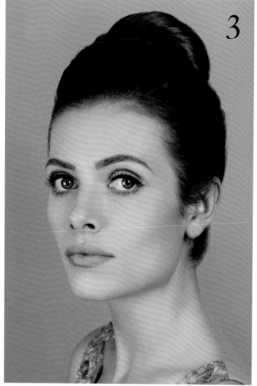

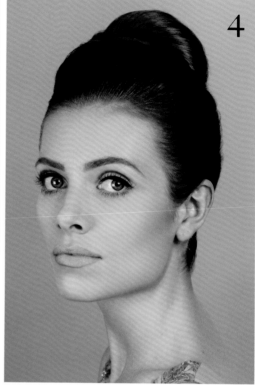

Step 3

Mascara: Apply black mascara liberally to both the top and bottom lashes.

Step 4

Blusher: Apply a pale, peachy pink powder blusher to the cheekbones.

Lipstick: Apply a pale peach matte lip colour using a lip brush. The lips are kept a natural shape and are neither over- nor underdrawn.

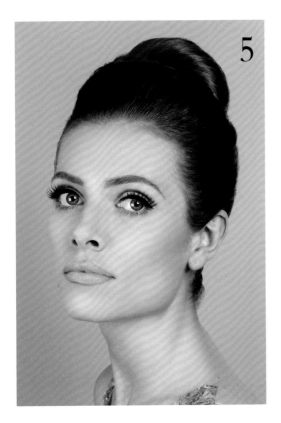

5

Step 5
Lashes: Trim strip lashes to the correct length and apply them to the upper lash line. I used medium-length false lashes for this look.

When it came to applying shadow, many people still used the sponge applicators that came with the colour, but some brands began to include better-quality brushes with their products.

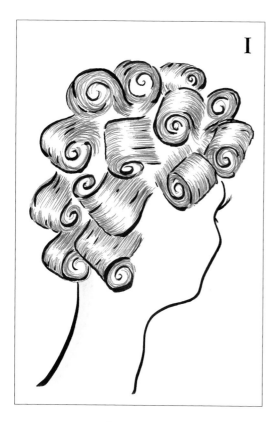

I

Step 1

This style is best achieved with a hairpiece, but if your own hair is thick and long enough, you can use plenty of backcombing and style it as described or go for a simpler version. The hairpiece Lou used here is made with wefted hair, about 8 x 8cm (3 x 3in) and 20cm (8in) long.

Set the hair and the separate hairpiece, if using, on large heated rollers, as shown above. You do not need a lot of curl for this style, so the number of rollers you use will depend on the length and thickness of the hair. When the rollers have cooled, remove them from both the hair and hairpiece.

Step 2

Put some serum on your hands and stroke through the hair, then take the hair up into a high ponytail just below the crown, making sure the hair going into it is nice and smooth.

Attach the hairpiece: you can either pull your own hair through it for extra security, or place it at the front of the crown, with your own hair behind it. Secure using hair pins.

Step 3

Divide the hair in sections about the same size and thickness as those on the hairpiece. If your own hair is not very long, you can hide it under the piece and simply use it to pin into.

Take a section of hair and backcomb the roots, then smooth into a petal shape, arrange in place and secure with hair grips (bobby pins). Work your way around the head, keeping an eye on the overall shape and blending your own hair in with the hairpiece.

For a shortcut to this look, just put your hair in a high ponytail and set the pony in a few rollers, then style as described above.

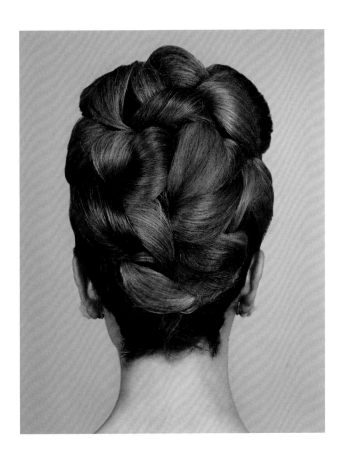

In the 1960s, it was very common for women to use hairpieces to enhance their styles.

This sophisticated 1960s look
can easily be adapted to suit
a variety of occasions.

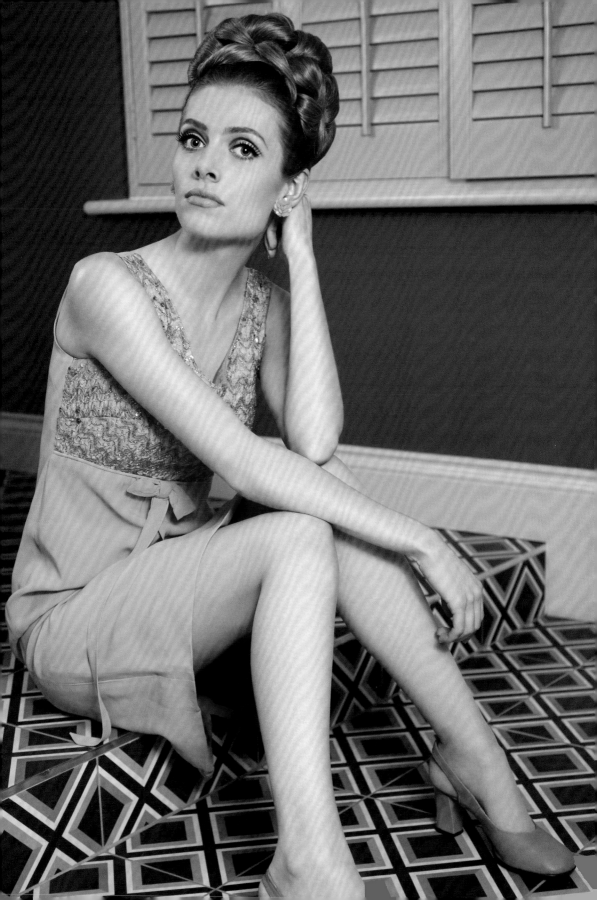

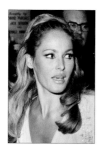

This look can be worn casually or in a more dressed-up way for the evening. The hairstyle is suitable for a range of hair lengths – our reference picture shows actress Ursula Andress wearing a long version. The make-up shown here is a variation on the classic defined socket line or 'cut crease' of Look 1 (see page 171), but I shaded the line up on to the brow bone slightly, still keeping the half-moon shape. Using black cake eyeliner and a fine liner brush, I painted on some eyelashes under the bottom lashes at the outer corners.

THE
—
1960S

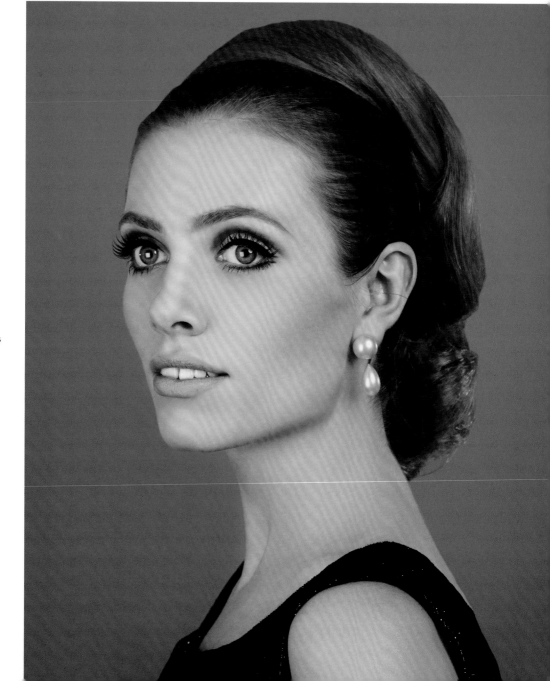

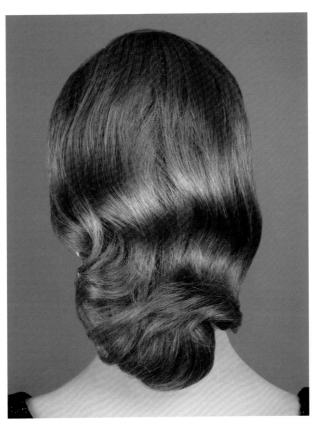

Hair

This hairstyle shows the
importance of a good set,
as it makes the styling much
easier and the finished look
more striking.

Set the hair on heated rollers
using the set shown in step 1
on page 174. When the rollers
have cooled, remove them.

Brush the hair up into a high
ponytail on top of the crown
and secure in a hairband.

Take a section of hair wide
enough to wrap around the
ponytail and wrap it loosely
around the base of the ponytail
to conceal the hairband. Secure
it with a few discreet hairgrips
(bobby pins).

This softer version of the classic 1960s 'cut crease' eye make-up is particularly suitable for those with hooded eyelids, as it 'lifts' the brow bone slightly.

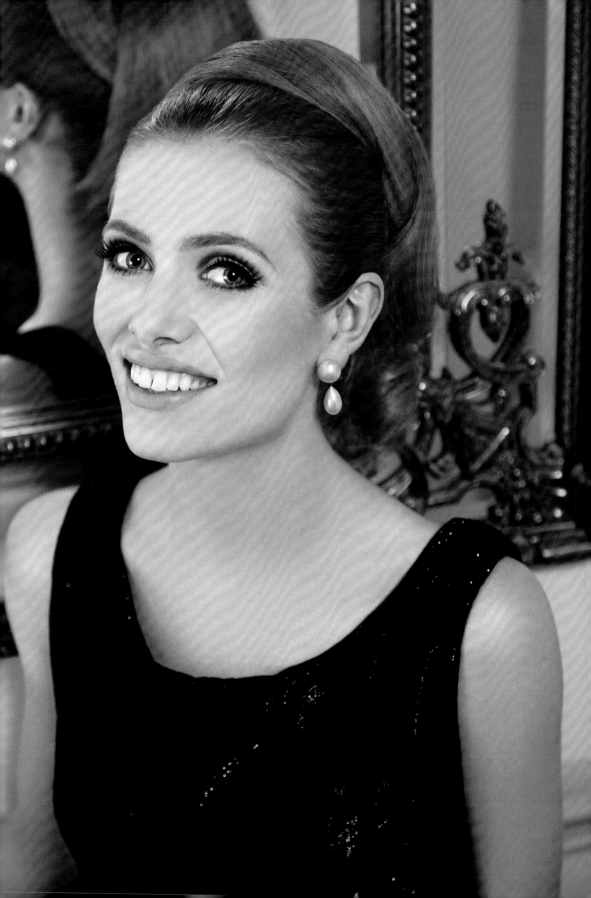

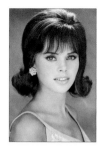

This look, with the flicked-up hair and heavy eyeliner, is what instantly springs to mind for many people when thinking of the 1960s style. Our reference picture of actress Britt Ekland shows a classic example of the look. Versions of this hairstyle were worn by women of all ages, making it one of the key shapes of the decade. As for the make-up, Max Factor's Pan-Stik foundation, which gave full coverage, was still very popular at this time, but some women wore more natural-looking bases.

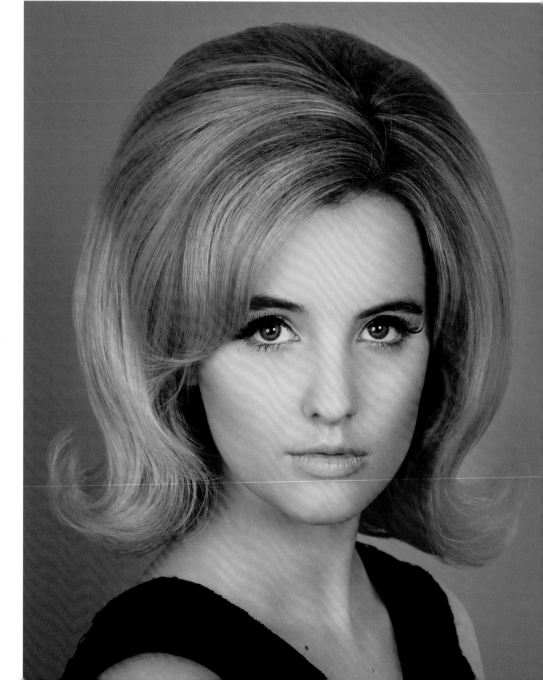

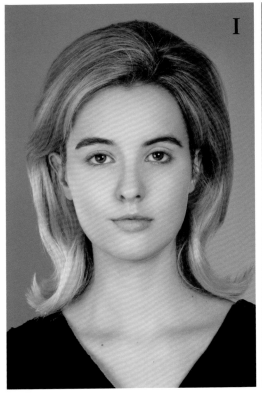

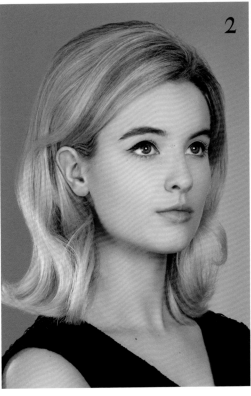

Step 1

Foundation: Apply foundation, followed by concealer and powder, as described in step 1 on page 19.

For the classic 1960s full-coverage look, I used a cream foundation here, matched exactly to the model's skin colour.

Step 2

Brows: The eyebrows are left natural and combed through.

Eyeshadow: Apply white matte powder shadow all over the lid and right up to the brow.

Eyeliner: Apply black cake eyeliner to the upper lash line using a fine brush. Make the line thickest at the middle of the eye and taper it to a point at the inner and outer corner. This makes the eyes look rounder, rather than the sweeping, elongated lines that make the eyes seem wider and further apart.

Mascara: Apply black mascara to both the top and bottom lashes.

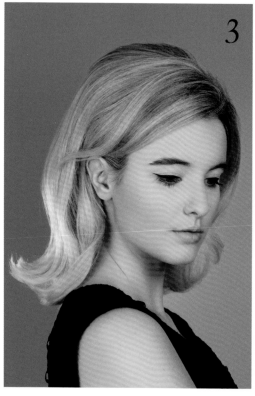

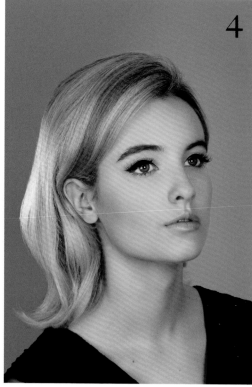

Step 3

Blusher: Using a blusher brush, apply powder blusher in a pale peach colour to the cheekbones.

Lightly shade under the cheekbones using a matte colour that is exactly the same tone as the natural shadows on the face – this is very important in order for the shading to look natural. Only apply the shading just under the cheekbones and do not take it down too far towards the centre of the face, as this will age you. The shaders that were used in the 1960s were a light brown or tan colour and didn't look natural.

Step 4

Lipstick: Apply a pale peach lipstick with a pearly finish.

Lashes: Add wispy-style false lashes only to the top lash line.

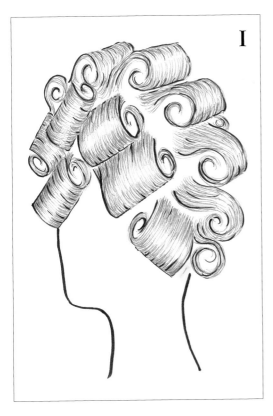

I

Step 1

Create a side parting, then set the hair, as shown above, using large heated rollers. To get the required volume, make sure the rollers are wound right to the roots of the hair.

Remove the rollers when they have completely cooled. Lightly brush the hair through.

To style, backcomb the hair at the roots, working all over the head. Then smooth the hair into the desired shape using a comb or a small brush, keeping the height. As you brush through, flick the hair up at the ends, controlling it with your hand.

Comb the front of the hair from the parting across the forehead, lifting it with a tail comb if you need more height.

Add hairspray to hold.

With added height at the crown and flicked-up ends, this is a key hairstyle of the 1960s.

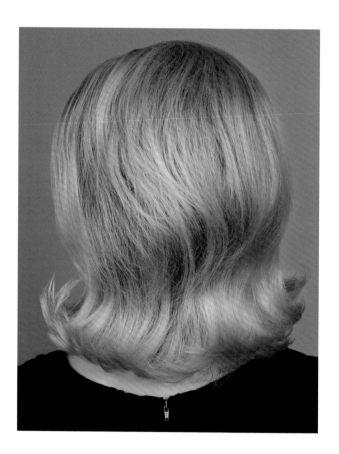

This is a classic 1960s style for day or evening. The lips are pale to keep the focus on the eyes – a trademark of the era.

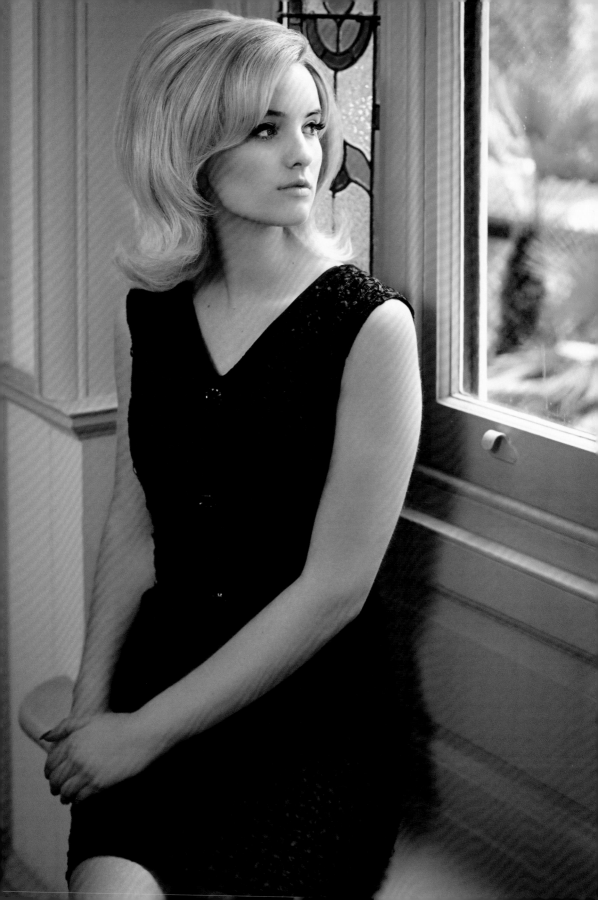

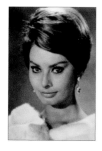

The beehive and variations on this look were widespread. Our reference picture shows Sophia Loren wearing a sophisticated evening version, whereas messier versions of this style could be seen on The Ronettes, one of the most popular girl groups of the 1960s, and more recently on another singer, the late Amy Winehouse. The elegant version shown here uses a French pleat at the back (see pages 146–9).

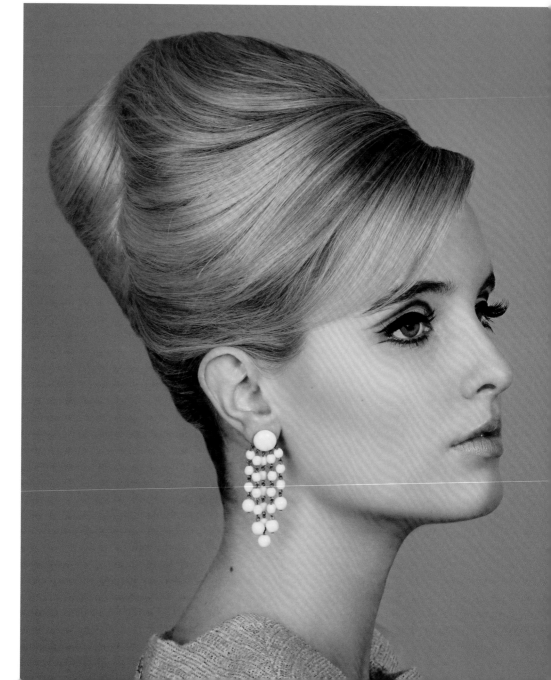

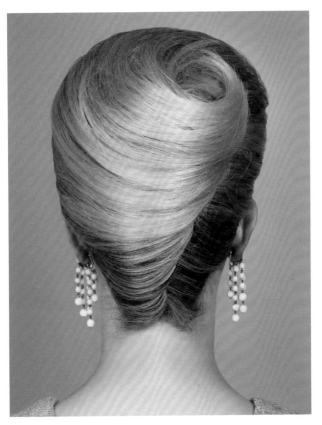

Make-up variation

Using black matte eyeshadow and a
pencil brush, draw a definite socket
line in the crease of the eye,
extending it out to the side and
tapering it to a point.

Apply black cake liner to the
upper lash line with a fine brush,
and flick it out slightly at the
outer corner.

Using the same brush and black
eyeshadow, draw a definite line under
the eye, winging it out to a point,
parallel to the end of the socket line.

Apply mascara, blusher and lipstick
as described on page 172.

Hair

Set the hair on heated rollers, as
described on page 185. Remove the
rollers when they have cooled and
lightly brush through.

Backcomb the hair all over to create
height, then smooth the surface,
using a little serum in your palm.

Create the French pleat as described
on page 147, but form more of a
'tornado' shape with a swirl at the top.

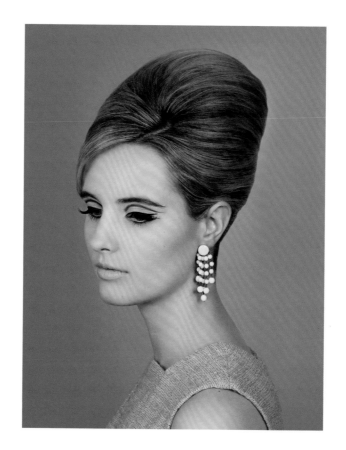

A chic, sleek, full-on 1960s
look that has been an
inspiration for fashion
lovers ever since.

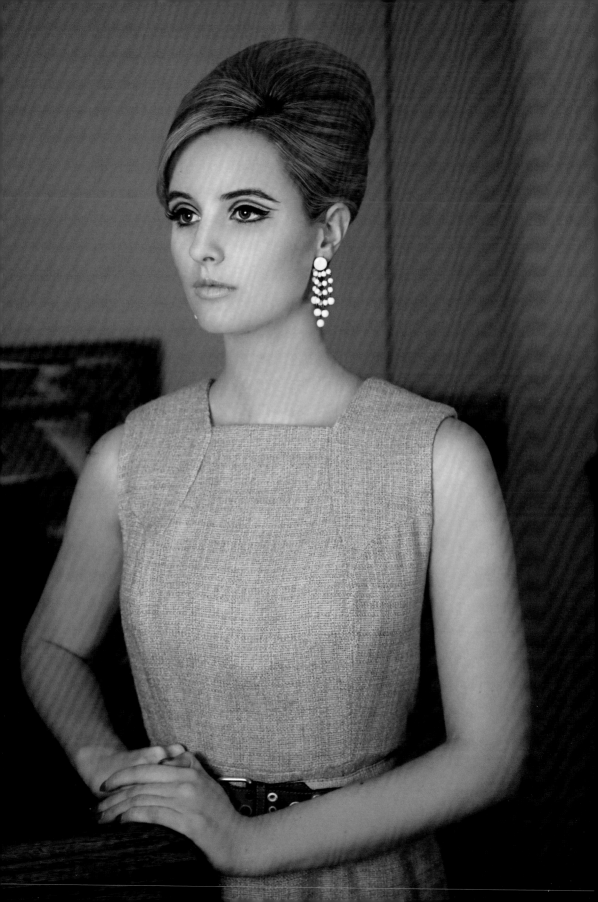

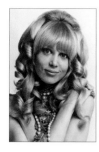

The 'baby doll' look was very popular during the 1960s. There was nothing natural about it, with extra-long false lashes used to give that wide-eyed and innocent look. Women often used hairpieces to add length and volume to this type of hairstyle, and also to transform a daytime look into an evening one. This glamorous style was seen on actress Raquel Welch and model Pattie Boyd (pictured here), among others. A much messier version was often worn by Brigitte Bardot.

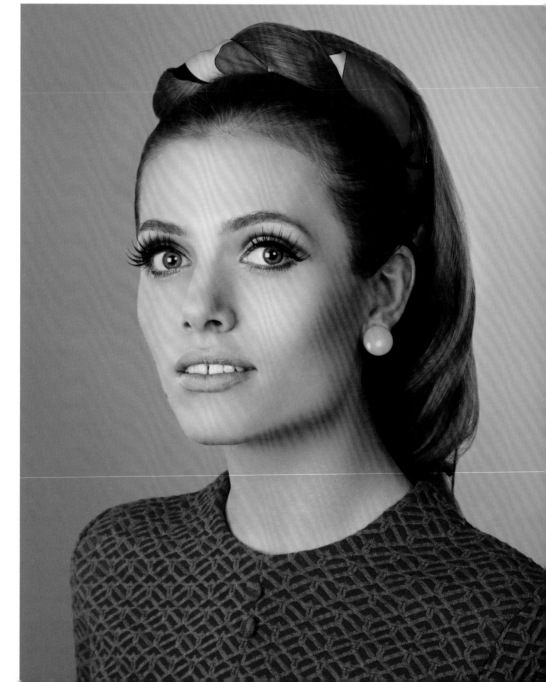

THE

1960S

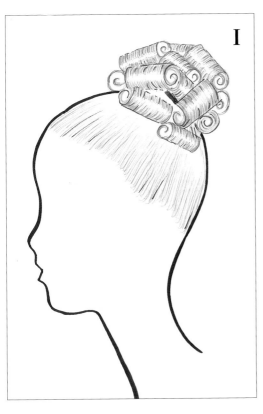

Make-up variation

This is a variation on Look 1, shown on page 170.

Shade above the definite socket line with a matte eyeshadow. I chose a rust colour, to match the model's dress.

As in Look 3, shown on page 184, I applied a little blush to the cheeks and a natural shader under the cheekbones.

The lip colour consists of concealer mixed with a pinky brown lipstick.

Apply black mascara to the top and bottom lashes, then complete this glamorous look with extra-long eyelashes applied to the upper lashes.

Hair

Secure the hair in a high ponytail and set the length with heated rollers, as shown above. At the same time, set a separate hairpiece with heated rollers to curl it. (If you have very thick, long hair, you can do this style without a hairpiece, simply using backcombing to add volume.)

Remove the rollers when they have completely cooled. Attach the curled hairpiece using the base of the ponytail as an anchor point.

Gently brush through the waves and let them fall in a waterfall effect.

To finish the look, choose a silk scarf that co-ordinates with the dress. Twist it around a section of hair and wrap it around the head. Tie the scarf at the back of the head, under the hair, using it to disguise the join of the hairpiece.

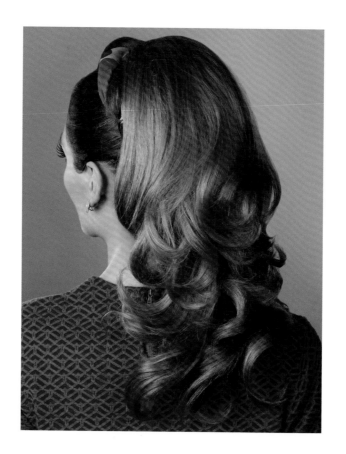

If you have a lot of hair,
you can do this style without a
hairpiece. Use backcombing
to add extra volume.

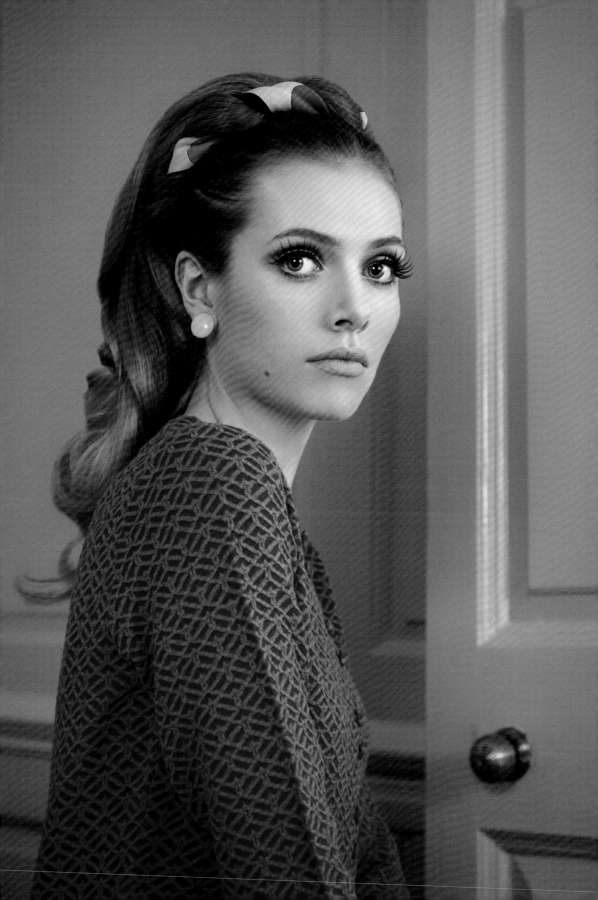

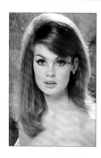

This is a much looser, less stiff 1960s style that can be adapted for a messier version as well. Our reference image shows Jean Shrimpton, one of the most famous faces of the decade. One of the world's great supermodels, she came to represent the epitome of the London It Girl, with her big, dramatic eyes and her miniskirts. The iconic photographs of Shrimpton taken by David Bailey, her partner at the time, helped propel both of them to fame and summed up the Swinging London of the 1960s.

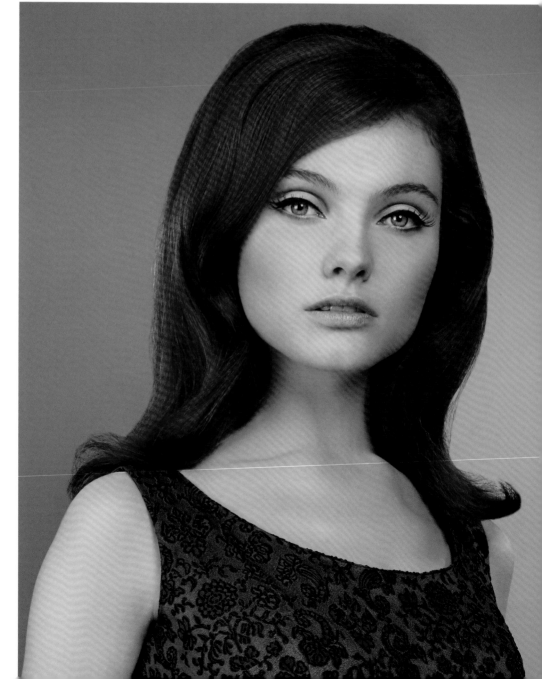

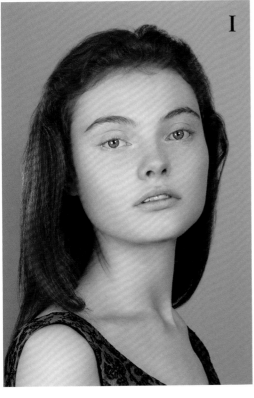

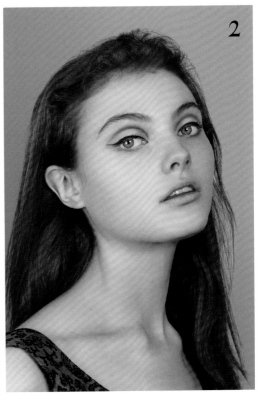

Step 1

Foundation: Apply foundation and concealer as described in step 1 on page 19.

Powder: Apply colourless loose powder all over the face using a puff and then dust off the excess with a powder brush. Apply the powder very lightly to allow the natural skin texture to show through.

Step 2

Brows: Fill in any gaps in the brows. I used a rust-coloured matte eyeshadow mixed with a little brown shadow to match our model's hair.

Eyeshadow: Apply white pearly eyeshadow over the lid. Use a pencil brush to apply a soft line of black matte shadow in the socket crease and under the eye.

Eyeliner: Using a fine eyeliner brush, apply black cake eyeliner only to the top lash line, winging it outwards and upwards at the outer corners and tapering it to a point.

Macara: Apply black mascara to the the top and bottom lashes.

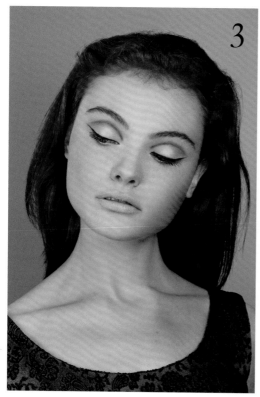

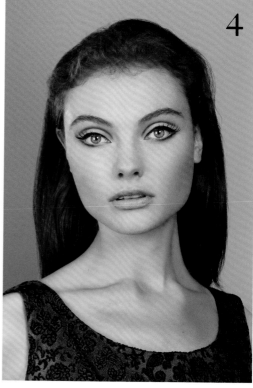

Step 3

Blusher: Brush a peach-coloured powder blusher over the cheekbones.

Step 4

Lipstick: Apply peach pearly lip colour using a lip brush.

Lashes: Add spiky black false lashes to complete the look.

Towards the end of the 1960s, young women started drawing on freckles with brown eye pencil – of course, only some girls followed this trend.

A longer version of the flick shown in Look 3 on page 182, this style could be made even more youthful by backcombing and ruffling the hair for a tousled effect.

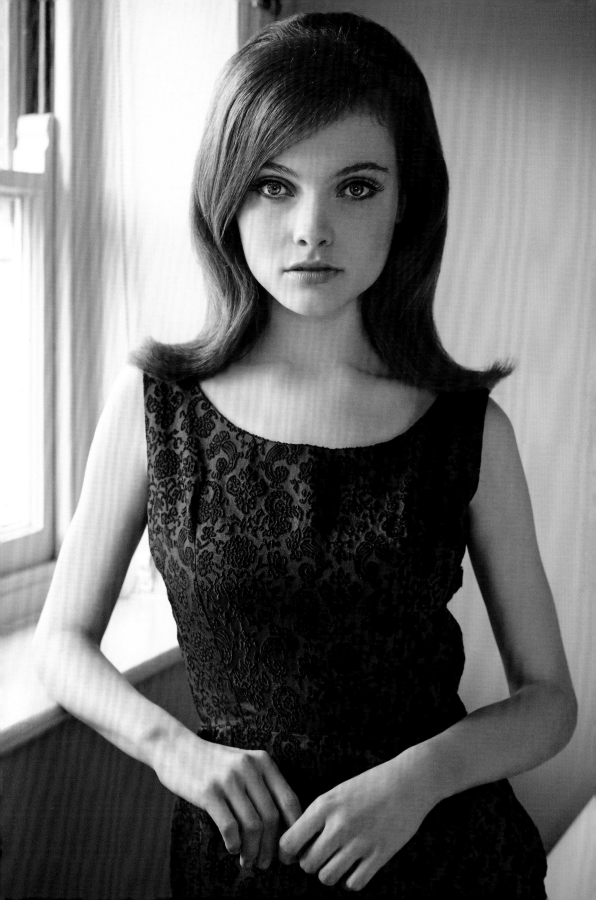

The 1970s

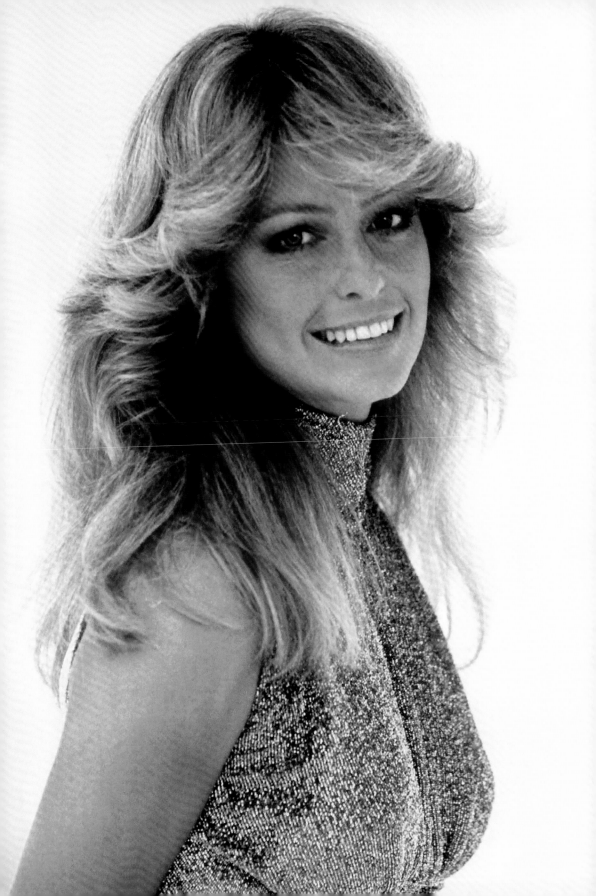

The 1970s

FROM GLAM ROCK TO PUNK AND EVERYTHING IN BETWEEN, IN THIS DECADE OF VISUAL AND MUSICAL EXTREMES, MAKE-UP, HAIR AND FASHION WERE INEXTRICABLY LINKED.

Whether it was flares and tank tops or the glitter of disco, there was something for everyone in the looks of the 1970s.

MAKE-UP

At the start of the decade the influence of bands such as Abba, T-Rex and Roxy Music led to a looser, more relaxed look in make-up. Girls often wore one colour of eyeshadow with glossy lips and blusher. Some men, from Marc Bolan to David Bowie in his Ziggy Stardust guise, started wearing make-up.

Offering an alternative to those polished, wholesome looks, the images photographer Sarah Moon created for Biba in the early 1970s harked back to the 1920s, featuring moody, romantic make-up. Revlon's Charlie perfume was launched in 1973, promoted with the image of the free-spirited young woman about town, and was soon followed by a Charlie range of make-up.

Max Factor continued to be a major player in the cosmetics industry, launching the Maxi range in the late 1970s. Aimed at the younger end of the market, it was intended to rival other youth brands Cover Girl and Charlie.

Then came the explosion that was punk: a heady period in 1977 when all the style rules were broken. From multiple piercings to 'tramlines' shaved into the hair, from the gothic extremes of Siouxie Soux's make-up to the Monroe-meets-punk glamour of lead singer Debbie Harry, innovative street styles emerged. Although short lived, the initial punk music scene left a lasting impression on hair and make-up styles.

By the end of 1977, fashion had begun to embrace elements of the punk style and, somewhat ironically, what had started out as a rebellion gradually became part of mainstream popular culture.

HAIR

During the late 1960s, longer, more natural hairstyles had become popular. Women of colour teased their hair into Afro styles, rather than straightening it – a look that reached its peak during the 1970s disco era.

By the start of the 1970s, with the rock scene influencing both women's and men's hair fashions, the more 'done', stiff styles of the mid-1960s became a thing of the past. The early 1970s saw long, flowing styles, often with a centre parting and sometimes with a fringe flicked back. Pageboys and halo-style demi waves and perms were popular, along with some styles that are best forgotten! The television show *Charlie's Angels*, starring Farrah Fawcett, started airing in 1976, and her glamorous waved hairstyle was soon copied the world over.

The 1977 film *Saturday Night Fever* cemented the disco revolution. New York's Studio 54 nightclub was frequented by film and music stars sporting an array of styles, from Jerry Hall's and Diana Ross's long curly locks to Grace Jones's severe crop.

The look of the glossy, all-American woman was in complete contrast to the punk styles that emerged in late 1976. At first, the spiky, dyed hair, Mohicans and shaved heads seemed shocking, but soon some of the punk-led techniques became mainstream.

Opposite: Farrah Fawcett, 1976

A number of looks were fashionable in the 1970s, but the predominant themes that ran through the cosmetics of the decade were gloss and shine. Women could choose from a vast array of products and textures in their continuing quest for glowing, tanned beauty. Leading brands were Revlon, Max Factor, Yardley, Maybelline, Estée Lauder, Elizabeth Arden and Helena Rubinstein. Mary Quant and Biba offered a youthful, very different colour range.

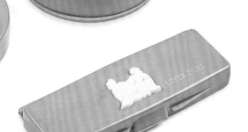

▼ Mary Quant foundation

In 1972, Mary Quant launched her Special Recipe range, which focused on the use of natural, pure ingredients. This tapped into the growing interest in natural products during the era.

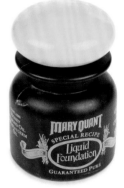

▲ Geminesse powder, compact and cake liner

Max Factor's high-end Geminesse range was packaged in Grecian-inspired containers. It featured beautiful ultra-frosted eyeshadows and lipsticks, and even frosted cream foundations and, to go over them, frosted loose powders, which gave a luminous appearance to the skin. The range was very expensive compared with most cosmetics available at the time.

Biba shampoo ▶

Herbal recipes or products that sound 'pure' and 'natural', such as these three Biba shampoos, boasting ingredients such as rosemary and lemon, were very popular in the early 1970s.

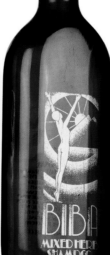
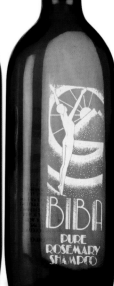

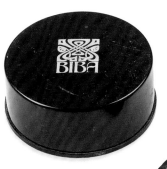

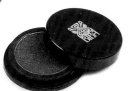

Biba eyeshadow ▼ ▶

Dark, dramatic shades such as plum or navy blue were key to the Biba look, worn with matching lipstick and blusher.

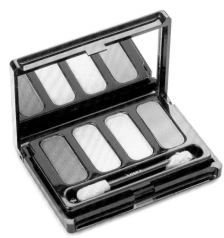

Biba loose powder ▲

The distinctive packaging of Biba make-up products was in line with the glitzy Art Deco style of the brand's flagship London store.

Mary Quant Special Recipe lipstick ▶

Advertisements for this Special Recipe range featured the make-up products photographed among various fresh vegetables, thus promoting the natural ingredients theme.

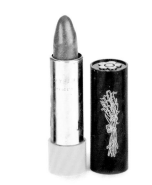

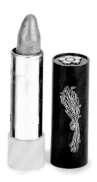

◀ Biba paintbox

Dating from the early 1970s, this set features products such as Face Gloss, Watercolour eyeliners, Contour Powder and Powder Tint shadows.

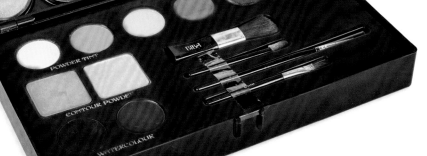

Max Factor's Geminesse range featured Rainbow Blue eyeshadow and Rich Pinkpenny Frost lip colour, which gives an indication of the colourful, frosty looks in favour at the time. Geminesse also featured some matte shadows, though these were never as popular as the high-gleam shades of the late 1970s. For many years Flori Roberts (launched in 1965) and Fashion Fair (launched in 1973) were the go-to brands for women of colour, until major companies finally introduced darker tones to their foundation ranges.

LIPSTICK

Roll-on, flavoured lip glosses were available in the early 1970s, when often a fairly natural lip would be worn in the daytime – either clear or natural and usually glossy. Stronger colours were worn in the evening, ranging from red to plum and more earthy tans and corals, all topped off with gloss.

EYESHADOW

A single colour was often worn on the lids and there was an array of hues to choose from – pale blue, turquoise, lilac, sea green and shades of brown. The early 1970s did not see the sophistication of application of the next decade, and there were some strange, unflattering looks advocated by magazines, including rainbow stripes of different colours across the eyelids. Biba and Mary Quant offered darker, moodier shadows than the more mainstream cosmetics companies.

BLUSHER

Highlighters were used to give a natural sheen, along with either cream or powder blushers. Tawny was a popular shade of blusher. The words 'natural', 'healthy', 'glow' and 'bringing out the best in you' were often used in cosmetics advertising, which gives a feel of the type of looks being promoted.

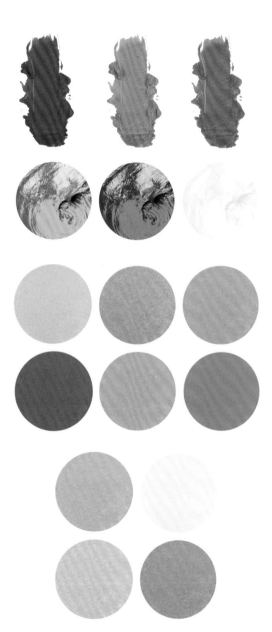

The strong colours of the punk scene were a direct contrast to the frosted pastels of mainstream make-up.

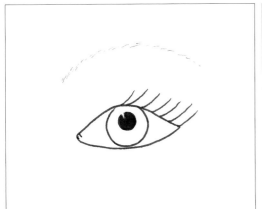

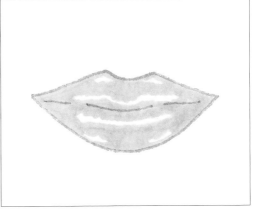

Brows

In the early and mid-1970s, many women really overplucked their eyebrows. Sometimes the brows never recovered from this repeated removal and, when thicker eyebrows came into fashion in subsequent decades, many women rued the day they started opting for the ultra-thin brow (shown above).

Later in the 1970s it became fashionable for brows to be left a little fuller, heading towards the superbrows of the 1980s.

Lips

Glossy, natural lips were worn during the day and glossy, more vibrant colours in the evening.

In complete contrast to the glossy, natural, girl-about-town looks that most cosmetics companies catered for, Biba lipsticks came in colours such as dark green, navy blue, pale blue, yellow, purple and fuchsia pink.

Tans were in fashion, and some women sunbathed to excess. Fake tanning products were available, as was make-up to enhance the glossy, suntanned look.

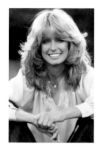

One of the classic 1970s looks that many women tried to emulate was The Farrah, named after the actress Farrah Fawcett (pictured), one of the stars of the popular American TV series *Charlie's Angels*. Her blonde mane, tumbling in soft waves and flicks over her shoulders, prompted girls all over the world to reach for their heated rollers. Farrah embodied the glossy, wholesome, all-American look that was the height of fashion at the time, and this hair and make-up style was copied by women everywhere.

THE

1970S

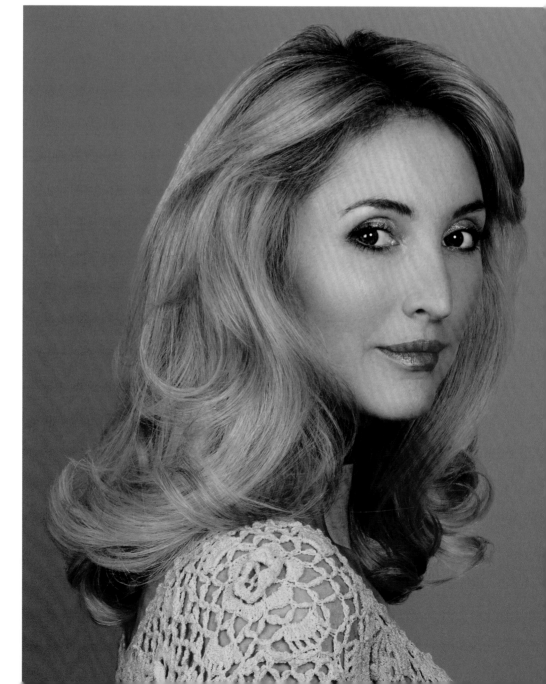

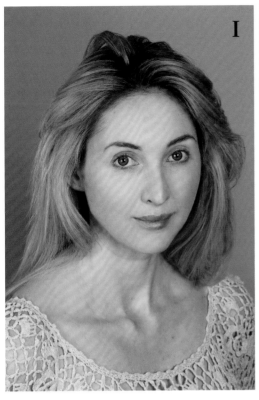

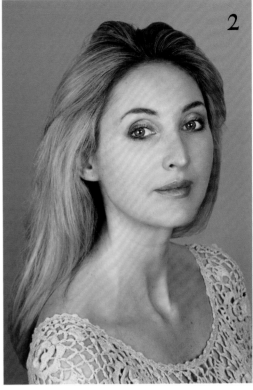

Step 1

Foundation: This look requires the foundation to look as natural as possible, so choose a light, sheer liquid foundation or a tinted moisturizer. Match it to the skin colour, mixing two shades together if necessary, and apply with a brush as described in step 1 on page 19.

Concealer: Using a concealer brush, apply a lighter shade on any dark areas under the eyes and a shade that matches the foundation on any blemishes on the face.

Powder: Apply a very light dusting of loose powder using a powder brush. This lets the natural sheen of the skin shine through the make-up.

Step 2

Brows: Keep the eyebrows natural and just brush them through with a mascara brush. If necessary, lightly fill in any gaps using matte brow powder or eyeshadow in a shade that matches the natural brows.

Eyeshadow: Apply pastel-pink shimmery eyeshadow over the lid and up to the socket crease. Then add a soft, matte purple in the outer corner of the eye.

Eyeliner: Apply matte purple shadow under the outer two-thirds of bottom lashes.

Mascara: Apply black mascara to the top and bottom lashes.

Lashes: Sometimes false lashes were used for an evening look, but they were more wispy and natural-looking than the ones worn in the 1960s.

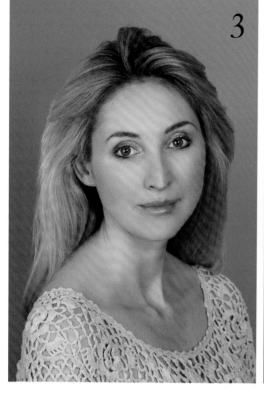

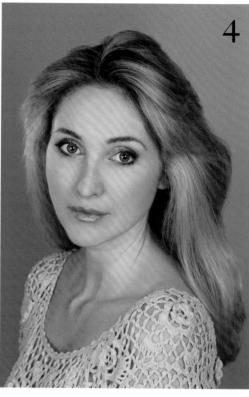

Step 3

Blusher: Blend a soft pink powder blusher over the cheekbones with a blusher brush.

Highlighter: Add a touch of shimmery powder highlighter along the top of the cheekbones with a soft brush to keep the look fresh and glowing.

Step 4

Lipstick: Apply lipstick in a shimmery pale pink to complete the look.

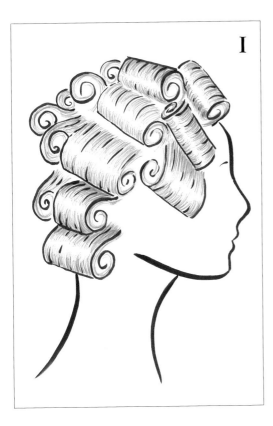

Step 1

Set the hair on large heated rollers, as shown above. Start at the front and work over the back of the head and down the sides, rolling the hair under and angling the side rollers slightly towards the back.

Remove the rollers when they have completely cooled.

To style, gently brush through the waves. A small amount of backcombing at the roots will give the hair extra volume.

This flattering, glamorous look is still relevant today and is quick and easy to achieve.

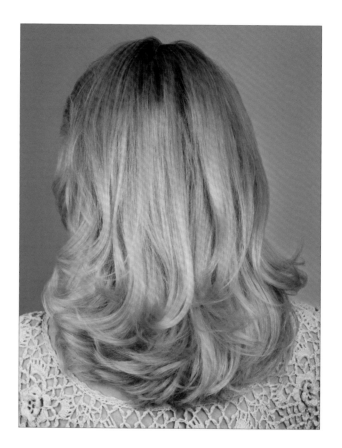

The look of the 1970s is softer
and glossier than that of the
previous decades.

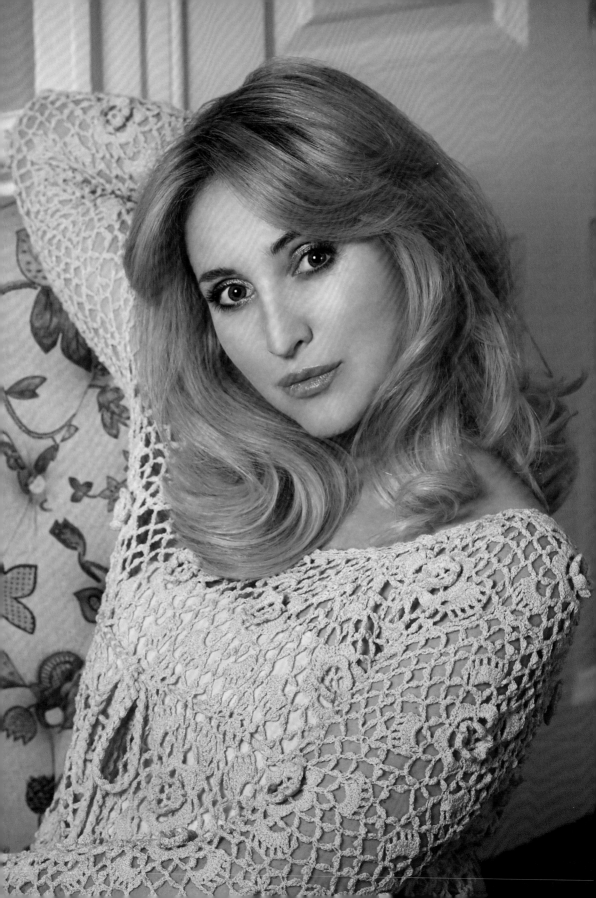

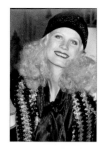

Biba girls were an alternative to all the fresh-faced, Californian girls-next-door during the 1970s and they inspired many looks, such as the one seen here in our reference image of the model Twiggy. This look was achieved in only ten minutes of make-up time and ten minutes of hairstyling, but it is one of my favourites in the book and I think it stands the test of time.

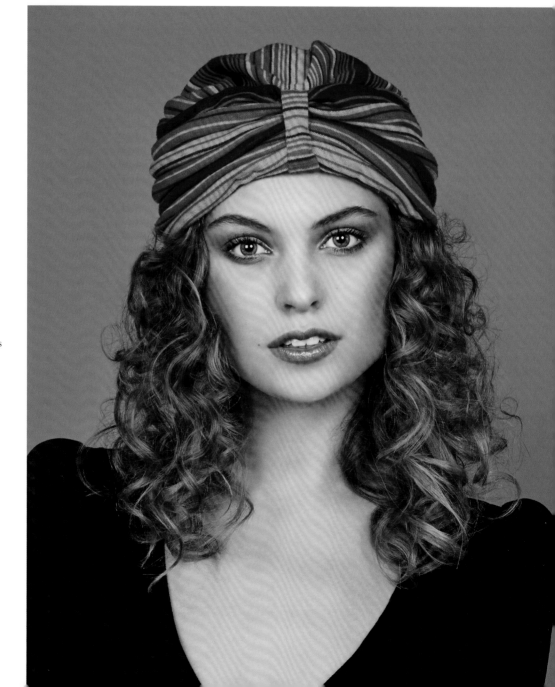

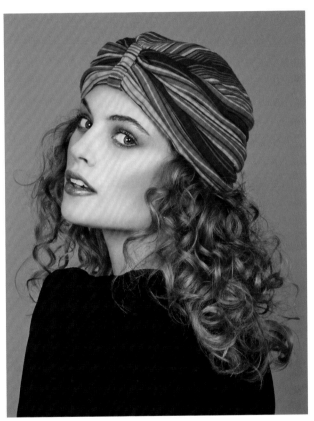

Make-up variation

Apply foundation, concealer and powder as in Look 1 (see step 1, page 211).

Leave the brows in their natural shape and just brush them through.

The eye, cheek and lip make-up here was all done using one palette. Brush a copper/bronze shadow over the lids and under the lower lashes. Take the same product on to the cheeks for a healthy glow, and then mix the pigment with clear lip gloss to make the lip colour. Apply a dark green eyeshadow to the outer corners of the eyes to shape them. Blend the shadows out on to the temples to meet the blusher.

Apply black mascara to the top and bottom lashes.

Hair

Curl the hair with hot sticks, placing them in random directions to create maximum volume and curls. When they have cooled, take them out and let the hair fall into natural curls.

Turbans were very popular in the 1970s, both as daywear and for the evening, when more glitzy versions were worn. They're perfect for quick, fuss-free styles like this one.

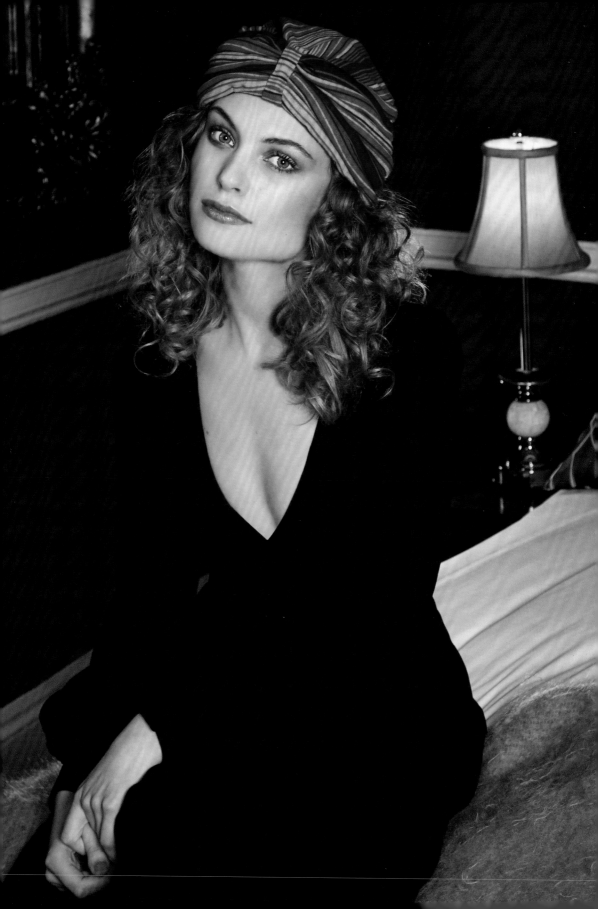

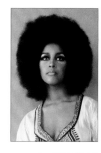

Disco fever was a worldwide phenomenon in the 1970s, influencing everything from fashion to hair and make-up styles. People went out to dance and to be seen and, for many, it is the images of inside Studio 54 from the late 1970s that sum up the disco era. The renowned New York nightclub, which opened in 1977, saw top models and celebrities show off their moves, and everyone from Andy Warhol to Michael Jackson, Mick Jagger and Jerry Hall to Grace Jones and David Bowie was spotted in the glamorous venue. The reference for this look is the beautiful actress Marsha Hunt.

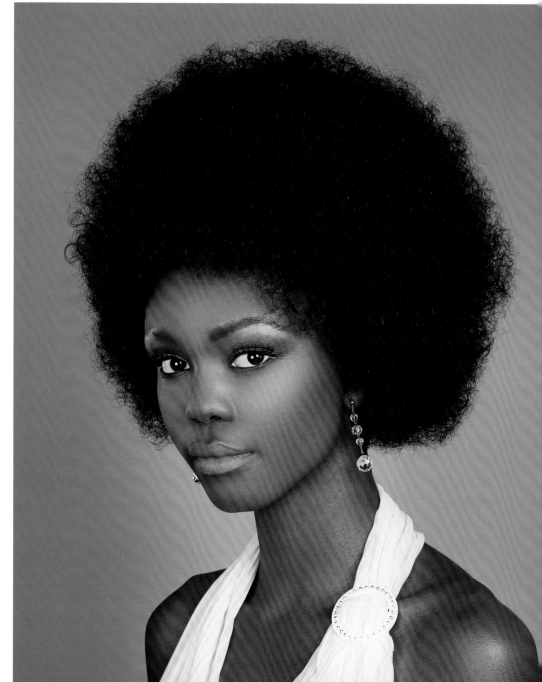

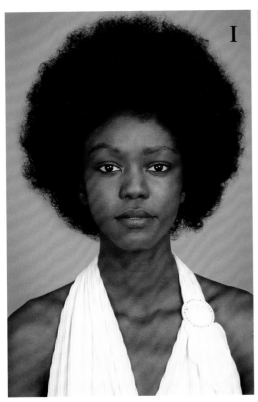

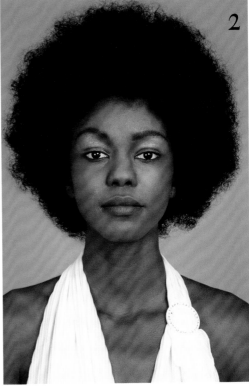

Step 1

Foundation: Use a liquid foundation for this look, matching it exactly to the skin tone; if necessary, mix two colours together to achieve a perfect match. Apply the foundation as described in step 1 on page 19.

Concealer: Apply concealer using a brush. Use a shade that matches the foundation to conceal blemishes and to even out pigmentation; use a lighter shade to cover up any dark shadows under the eyes.

Powder: Using a powder brush, apply fine colourless loose powder all over the face to set the make-up. Make sure the powder is absolutely colourless so it doesn't add colour but merely sets the make-up.

Step 2

Brows: Use a matte black/brown shadow and an angled brow brush to shape the brows into a gentle arch.

Eyeshadow: Apply a shimmering silver powder base colour all over the eyelid and up to the brow.

Apply a navy blue matte shadow on the socket crease and blend it upwards. Then brush the same colour under the lower lashes.

Mascara: Apply black mascara to the top and bottom lashes.

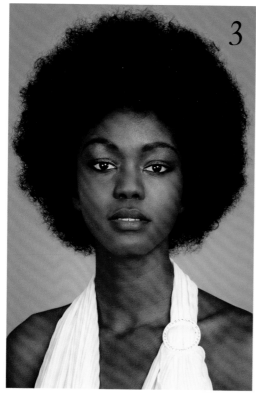

3

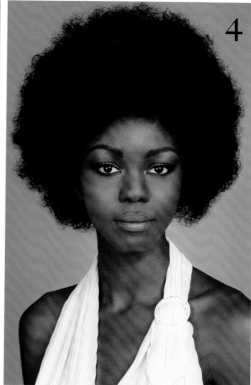

4

Step 3

Blusher: Apply a little russet-toned powder blusher to the cheekbones.

Step 4

Lipstick: Choose a lip pencil and a creamy matte lipstick in a colour that is a slightly lighter shade than the natural tone of the lips. Line the lips using the pencil and then fill in the shape with the lip colour using a lip brush.

Lashes: Apply full lashes to the top lids.

Eyeliner: Apply a dark navy liner on the top lashline to the conceal the join of the lashes.

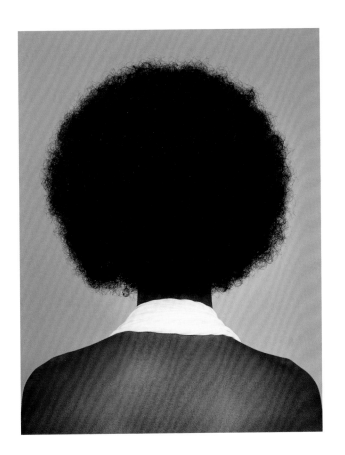

The hair was raked through
to shape and style the Afro, a style
that reached a peak of popularity
in the 1970s and was worn by both
men and women.

A classic look from the disco era, when dance music and the club scene had a strong influence on fashions in hair and make-up.

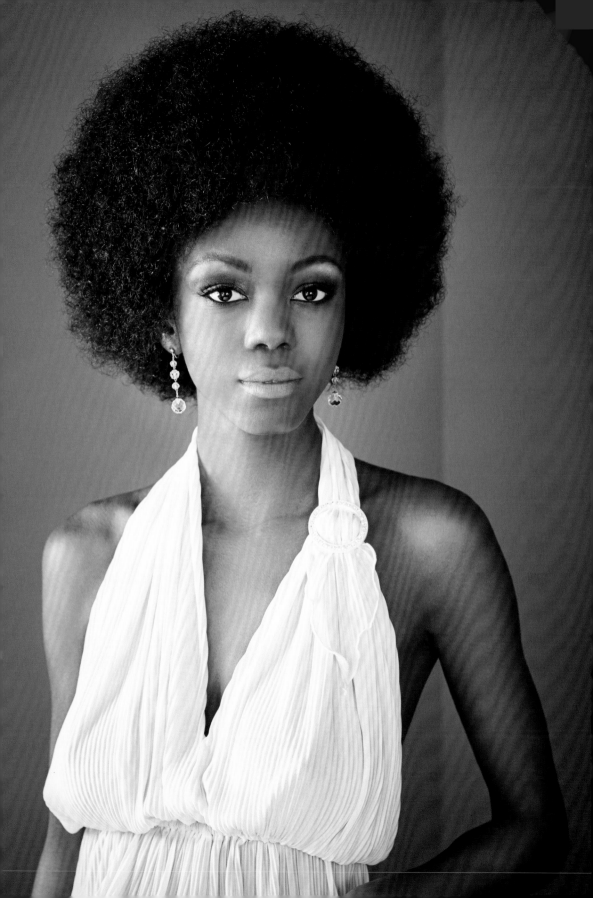

The 1980s and Beyond

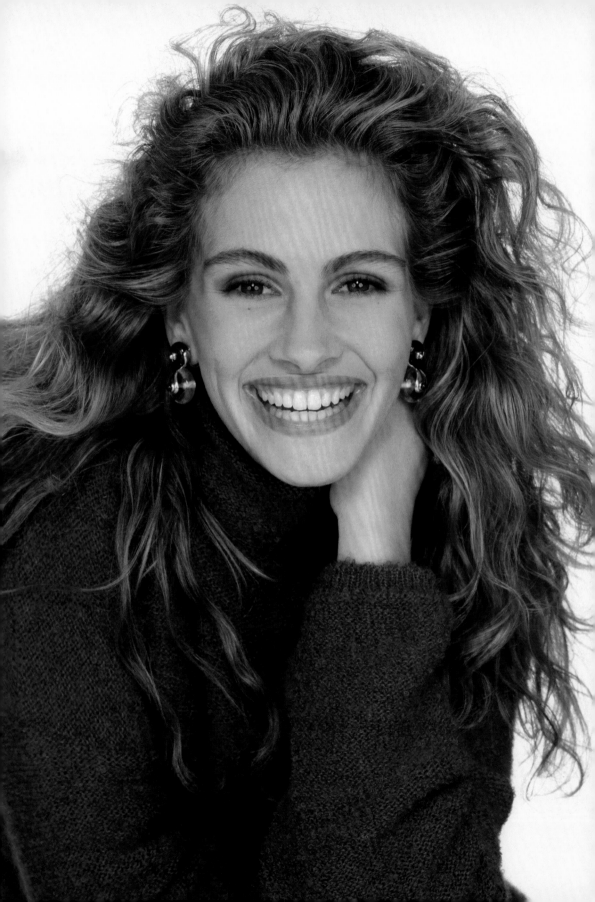

The 1980s and Beyond

THE CONTRASTING STYLES OF THE LATE 1970S PAVED THE WAY FOR THE COLOURFUL, ECLECTIC 1980S, A DECADE RESPONSIBLE FOR MANY CRIMES AGAINST FASHION BUT PROBABLY LOVED BY ALL IN SOME WAY. IN THE 1990S THINGS TOOK A TURN FOR THE MINIMAL AND MUTED.

1980s MAKE-UP

TV shows such as *Dallas* and *Dynasty* showcased power-dressing leading ladies with perfectly applied, dramatic make-up. Princess Diana became a style icon and her electric-blue eyeliner was much copied. Colourful, often clashing, eyeshadows were popular, worn blended up into the thick, unplucked eyebrows made famous by actress Brooke Shields. In the 1980s, dressing up was an art, with oversized tops, big hair and full make-up all essential.

In London clubs such as Blitz and Camden Palace the New Romantics took hair and make-up to another level, while in the USA Madonna burst on to the scene with her punk-inspired looks.

The late 1980s saw the rebirth of the supermodel – Christy, Linda, Claudia, Nadja, Cindy and Naomi personified the sexy, well-groomed, ultra-beautiful woman. Perfectly applied make-up in neutral colours heralded the advent of more subtle looks towards the end of the decade, with British *Elle* featuring a more natural-looking Yasmin Le Bon on the cover in 1985.

1980s HAIR

Probably the hottest hair trends in the 1980s were big hair and perms. Spiral perms, root perms, piggyback perms – everyone seemed to have one, including men. Other trends saw punk spikiness at the front, hair dyed a different colour, additions and false pieces. From shaved undercuts (a punk hangover) to extensions pioneered by London salon Antenna, hairstyles made a statement.

1990s MAKE-UP

A fresh-faced Kate Moss graced many magazine covers and advertising campaigns in the early 1990s. Clear skin, minimal make-up and nude colours were now the mainstream order of the day. In contrast, the grunge look featured smudgy kohl-ringed eyes, pale faces and dark-stained lips.

Bestselling products included Yves Saint Laurent's Touche Éclat (launched in 1991), Chanel's Rouge Noir nail varnish (launched in 1994), the sales of which skyrocketed after Uma Thurman wore it in *Pulp Fiction*. Brown lipstick was a key trend, with Rimmel's Heather Shimmer a favourite. MAC Cosmetics, founded in 1984, worked closely with the fashion and music industry, and grew to be one of the most successful make-up companies worldwide.

1990s HAIR

Jennifer Aniston's Rachel cut, named after her character from the TV series *Friends*, became one of the styles of the decade. Actress Meg Ryan's tousled blonde hair was another firm favourite.

The music scene saw Gwen Stefani sporting hair knots, quiffs, braids, cornrows and hair colours from bright pink to electric blue and platinum blonde. Crimping made a brief comeback and hair accessories such as butterfly clips and scrunchies were an essential part of many looks. The Spice Girls' carefully marketed image gave us partial pigtails (Baby), curls (Scary), long and natural (Sporty), backcombed glamour (Ginger) and sleek and well groomed (Posh) – something to appeal to every young fan.

Opposite: Julia Roberts, 1989

The make-up of the 1980s was an explosion of colour and textures. MTV launched in 1981, and in 1985 Robert Palmer's 'Addicted to Love' video featured models with slicked-back hair, heavily made-up dark eyes and glossy, red lips. After the excesses of the 1980s, the 1990s were more pared-down. In 1994, former model Iman launched her range of multi-ethnic colours, and as the decade progressed, major cosmetics brands followed suit, offering a wider range of shades.

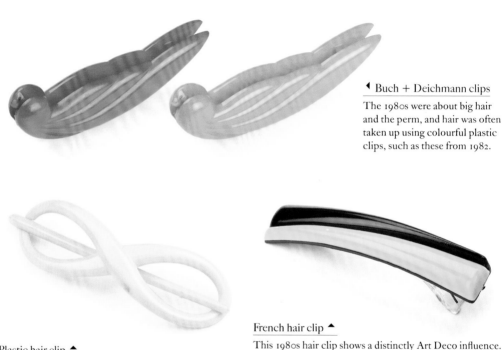

◀ Buch + Deichmann clips

The 1980s were about big hair and the perm, and hair was often taken up using colourful plastic clips, such as these from 1982.

French hair clip ▲

This 1980s hair clip shows a distinctly Art Deco influence.

Plastic hair clip ▲

Dating from 1981, this is a copy of a classic 1940s hair clip.

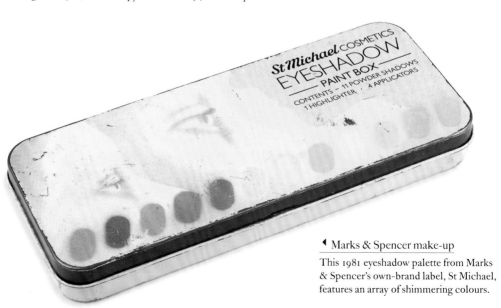

◀ Marks & Spencer make-up

This 1981 eyeshadow palette from Marks & Spencer's own-brand label, St Michael, features an array of shimmering colours.

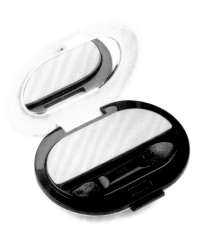

Revlon Ultima eyeshadow ▲

Revlon's Ultima brand was one of the first to sign an exclusive contract with a supermodel – Lauren Hutton This is an eyeshadow from the early 1980s.

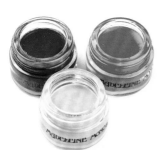

Madeleine Mono lip colour ▶

A collection of Madeleine Mono lip-colour pots, showing a range of colours including red, plum, orange and fuchsia.

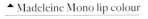

▲ Madeleine Mono lip colour

The range included a gold gloss, which was often added in the middle of the bottom lip over lipstick to create a pout.

Madeleine Mono blusher ▶

Brightly pigmented blushers from Madeleine Mono.

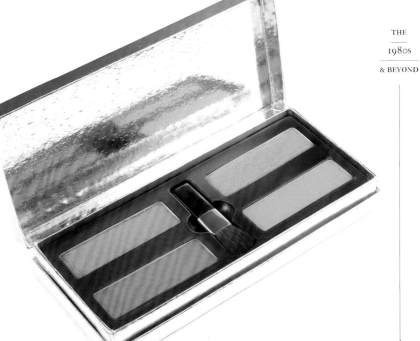

In the 1980s, women often used two, three or even four different eyeshadows at once, often in clashing colours – although some of these looks were very skilfully applied and perfectly blended. Brightly coloured eyeliner pencils, such as the electric blue worn by Princess Diana, were in fashion, and black, blue or teal pencil would often be used on the waterline. Bobbi Brown launched her range of nude lip colours in New York in 1991 – so very different from the brights of the previous decade, they set the tone for the colours of the 1990s.

The 1980s saw some extreme make-up looks, with bright colours used on lips, cheeks and eyes.

LIPSTICK

Popular lipstick colours in the 1980s were red, fuchsia, plum, russet, orange, frosted pinks and gold. In the 1990s nude and caramel-coloured lipsticks and glosses were popular, along with grungy maroons and plums.

EYESHADOW

Many different colours of eyeshadow were worn in the 1980s, and different textures were also available, including frost, matte and pearl. Popular colour combinations were pink/blue, gold/green, orange/teal and pink/grey. In the 1990s eyeshadows were mainly natural browns and creams, though purple was a trend for a while. A predominantly natural look was the way to go, other than the grunge trend, which brought black, kohl-ringed, smudgy eyes into fashion.

BLUSHER

In the 1980s highly pigmented blushers – some frosty and in electric colours – were worn, taken over the cheekbones and up on to the temples and hairline. Blusher was also used on the forehead and chin. In the 1990s brown and neutral blushers were favoured, while music-following grunge girls wore minimal blusher, as a pale face was the fashion.

THE

1980s

& BEYOND

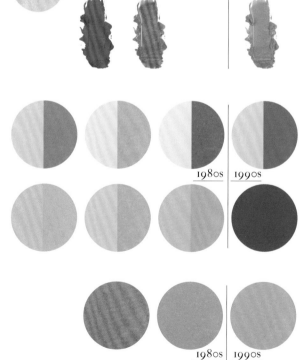

1980s | 1990s

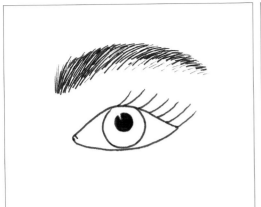

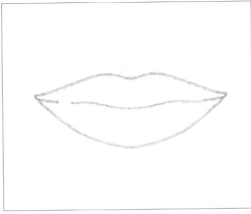

1980s Brows

In the 1980s, eyebrows were left natural and unplucked, and just brushed into shape.

1980s Lips

Full, colourful lips were in fashion, often glossy and sometimes overdrawn – although this can look very unnatural and is not a good look in real life.

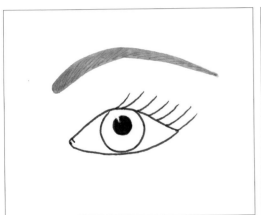

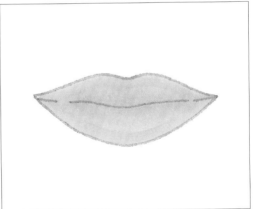

1990s Brows

A more groomed and shaped brow was popular in the 1990s – sometimes overplucked.

1990s Lips

Brown lips were very popular in the 1990s. Shades of raisin, coffee, mocha and caramel were worn, as well as russet, red, fuchsia and purple glosses.

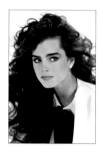

The 1980s were all about colour, big hair and big eyebrows, and this is a classic look from the decade, as worn by stars such as Julia Roberts and Brooke Shields (pictured left). The look works well with all the make-up colour combinations shown on page 232, so you can substitute different hues for the eyeshadows, blusher and lipstick. While singers such as Cyndi Lauper and Toyah Willcox flew the flag for more extreme 1980s looks, this is a style that was worn by many girls at the time and featured in many magazines.

THE

——

1980S

& BEYOND

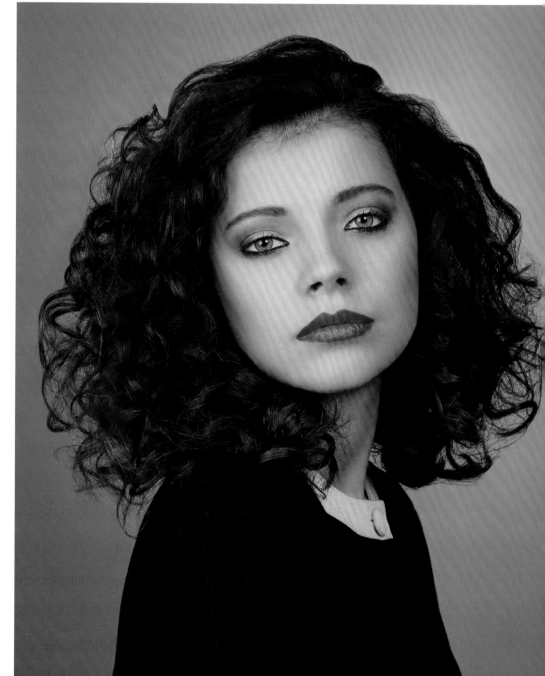

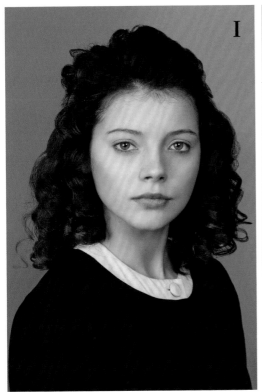

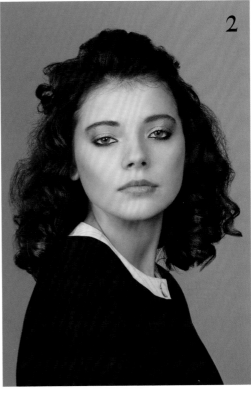

Step 1

Foundation: Apply foundation, followed by concealer and powder, as described in step 1 on page 19. You can add bronzer later if you wish to have more colour.

Step 2

Brows: Thicken the brows with matte eyeshadow, in a shade that matches the natural colour of your brows, using an angled brush. Then brush the brows upwards with a clean disposable mascara wand to achieve the desired fullness.

Eyeshadow: Apply a peachy pink frosted shadow all over the lid and up to the eyebrows. Apply russet/ brown matte shadow in the outer corner and into the socket crease. Using a fine brush, apply purple matte shadow under the eye, starting at the outer corner and fading it softly towards the inner corner.

Eyeliner: Fill in the bottom waterline using a black kohl pencil.

Mascara: Apply black mascara liberally to the top and bottom lashes. Coloured mascaras were popular in the 1980s and were available in purple, green and even orange.

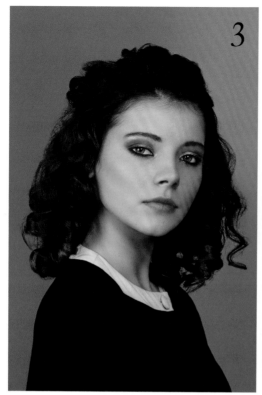

3

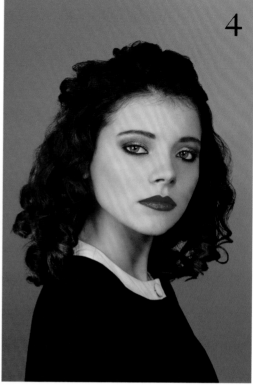

4

Step 3

Blusher: Using a blusher brush, apply red/rust blusher on the cheekbones and blend it outwards and into the hairline and upwards on to the temples.

Step 4

Lipstick: Line the lips with a bold red pencil and then use a lip brush to fill in the shape with a bright red lipstick.

Add a little gold shadow on the Cupid's bow of the top lip and in the centre of the bottom lip to catch the light and highlight the lips.

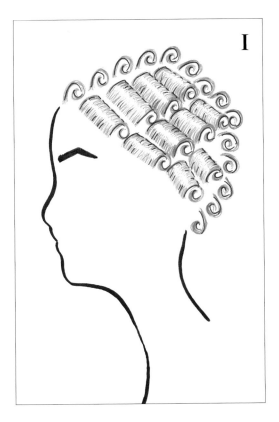

Step 1

Set the hair, as shown above, using small hot sticks (bendy rollers). Start at the centre front and work over the back of the head, winding the hair under. Then set the sides, rolling the hair away from the face and angling the hot sticks upwards and towards the crown.

After the hot sticks have cooled, remove them, and style the hair with your fingers to create the volume.

In the 1980s, hair would have been permed using small perming rods or curlers to get this look.

Scrunch-drying hair that has a natural wave gives a more tousled, messy look that was popular as well.

The big, curly hair, thick brows and multiple colours used on the face encapsulate the look and feel of the 1980s.

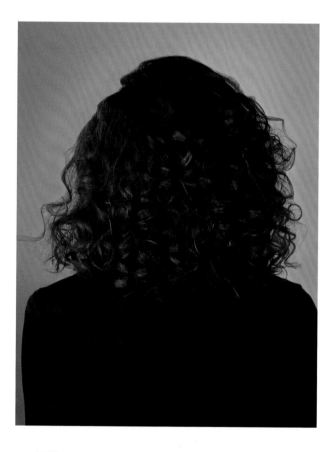

The constant perming and colouring of the hair often caused damage – and by the end of the 1980s, many women were happy to leave the permanent wave behind.

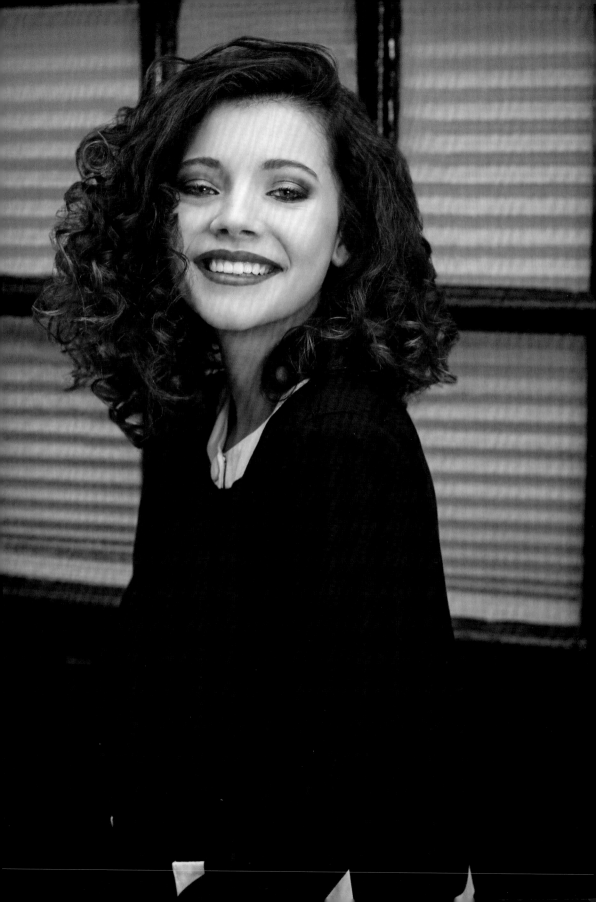

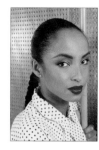

This elegant look is a pared-down version of some of the more extreme looks of the era. Our reference image here is of the singer Sade, whose understated (for the 1980s) style was much admired at the time. To achieve Sade's signature hairstyle, our model's hair was taken back into a small, flat bun and secured with a hairband. A switch was attached with pins, using the bun as an anchor point. Lou took a section of the switch and wrapped it around the join, then plaited the remaining hair on the switch.

THE

1980s

& BEYOND

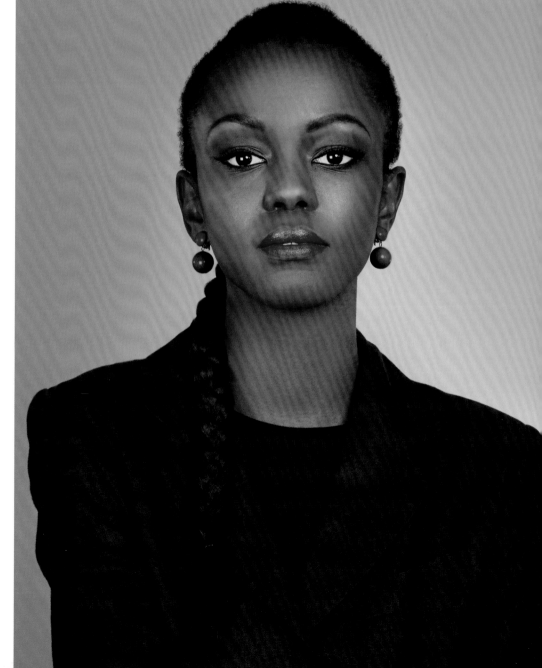

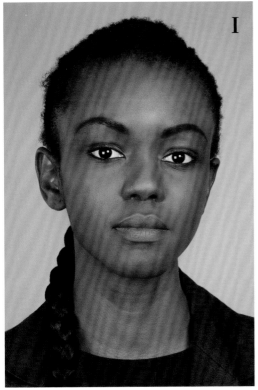

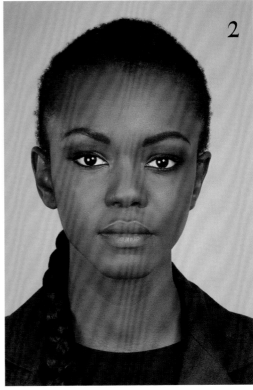

Step 1

Foundation: Apply foundation, followed by concealer and powder, as described in step 1 on page 19.

Brows: Make the eyebrows a little more groomed than in Look 1 (see step 2 on page 235). Apply a matching matte eyeshadow or brow powder to colour in and shape the brows, using an angled brush.

Step 2

Eyeshadow: Apply an orange/rust shadow as a base colour, brushing it over the lid and up to the brows. Apply dark brown matte shadow to the outer corner and blend it into and just above the socket crease. Apply black matte shadow under the eye, starting at the outer corner and blending it towards the inner corner.

Eyeliner: Apply black cake liner along the upper lash line, slightly elongating the line at the outer corner. Apply kohl pencil around the waterline.

Mascara: Apply black mascara to the top and bottom lashes.

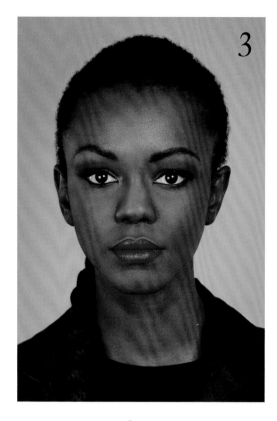

Step 3

Blusher: Apply russett-coloured matte powder blusher to the cheekbones.

Lipstick: Apply red lipstick with a creamy texture. No lip pencil was used for this look.

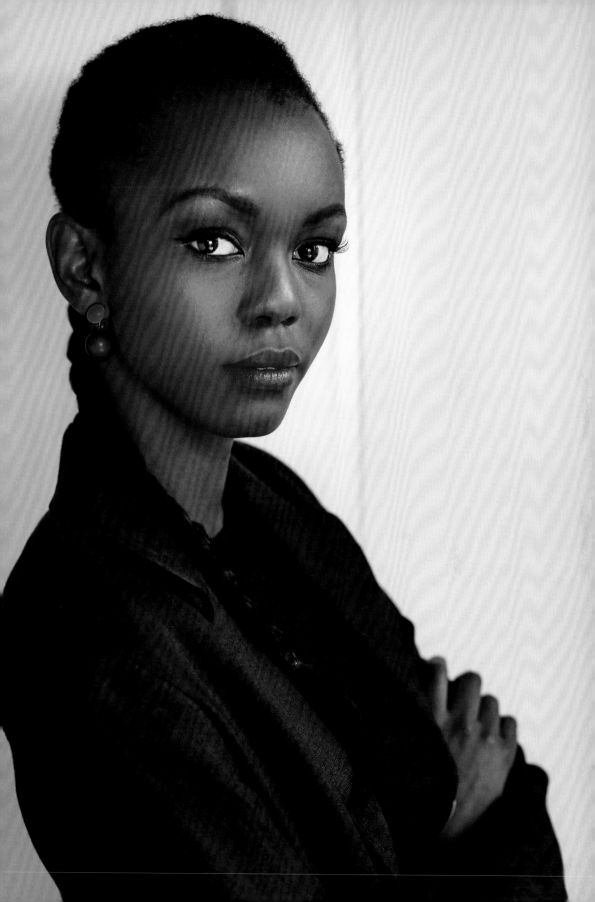

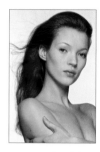

When we look back at the trends of the 20th century, we can see a pattern of extremes in make-up and hairstyles. After an extreme trend has reached its peak, we often see a move towards a much simpler style. The early 1990s are a great example of this: after the bright colours and big hair of the 1980s, the new decade ushered in more minimal trends for hair and make-up. This look is based on the make-up of the supermodels of the early 1990, such as Kate Moss (pictured) and Christy Turlington – a neutral, minimal look, that is easy to do and still chic today. Our model's straight hair was left natural.

THE

1980s

& BEYOND

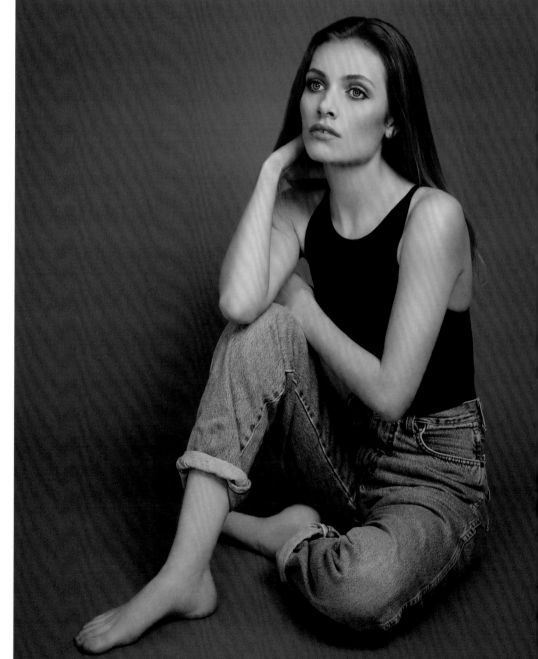

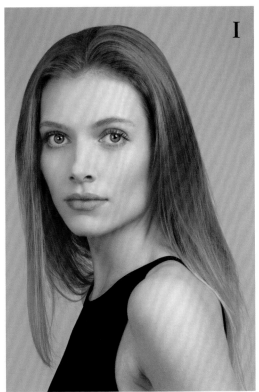

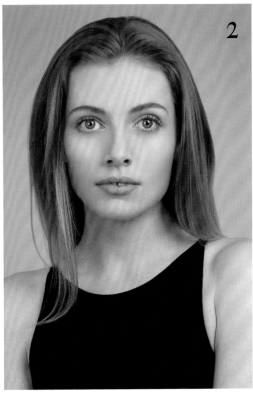

Step 1

Foundation: Apply foundation, followed by concealer and powder, as described in step 1 on page 19.

Step 2

Brows: Groom the brows using an eyebrow brush, adding a small amount of matching matte brow powder or eyeshadow where necessary to fill in any gaps.

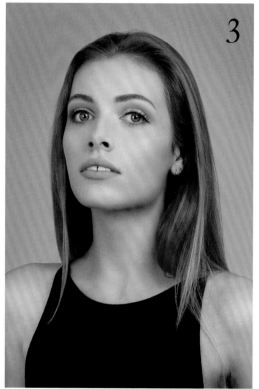

3

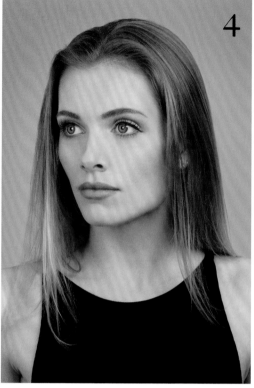

4

Step 3

Eyeshadow: Apply a neutral matte powder shadow to the lid as a base colour with a brush. Using a tapered shadow socket brush, lightly shade the socket line with a matte taupe shadow and blend onto the brow bone. Apply a small amount of the taupe shadow under the bottom lashes, fading out towards the inner eye corner. Make sure the shadow does not extend downwards at the outer corner of the eyes, as this is ageing and will make them appear to droop.

Eyeliner: Apply dark brown cake eyeliner along the upper lash line.

Mascara: Apply black mascara to the top and bottom lashes. Remove any clumps by combing them through with an eyelash comb.

Step 4

Blusher: Apply a muted soft brown/ peach blusher to the cheekbones with a blusher brush.

Lipstick: Apply a creamy lip colour in a nude, caramel shade, keeping the natural shape of the lips.

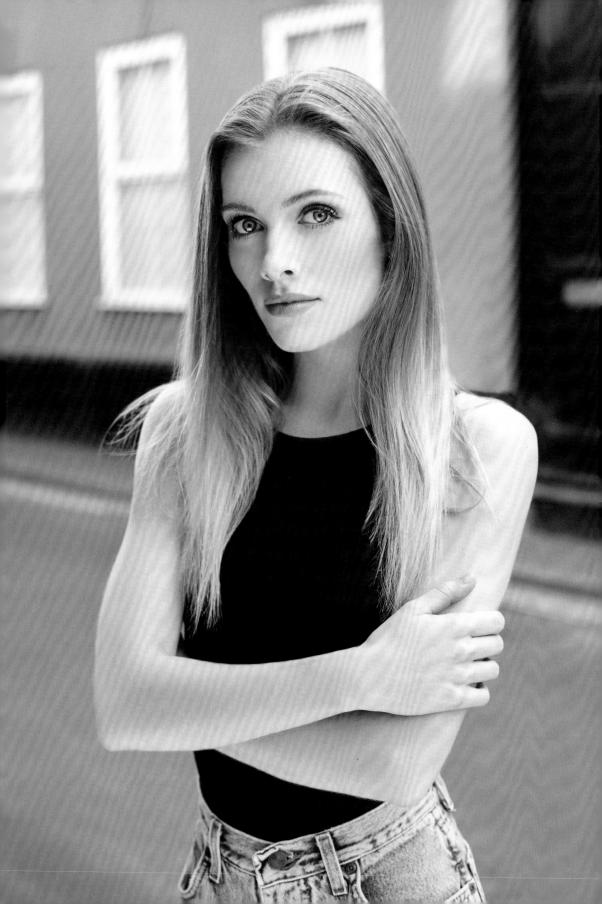

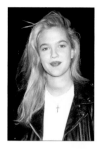

By the mid-1990s, grunge was at its height, thanks to the popularity of Seattle bands such as Nirvana and Soundgarden. The look was swiftly embraced by the fashion world and was soon seen on catwalks everywhere. Key elements of the look were unkempt hair and make-up that looked as if it had been slept in. Here, we are suggesting a slightly more polished version, as inspired by our reference picture of actress Drew Barrymore.

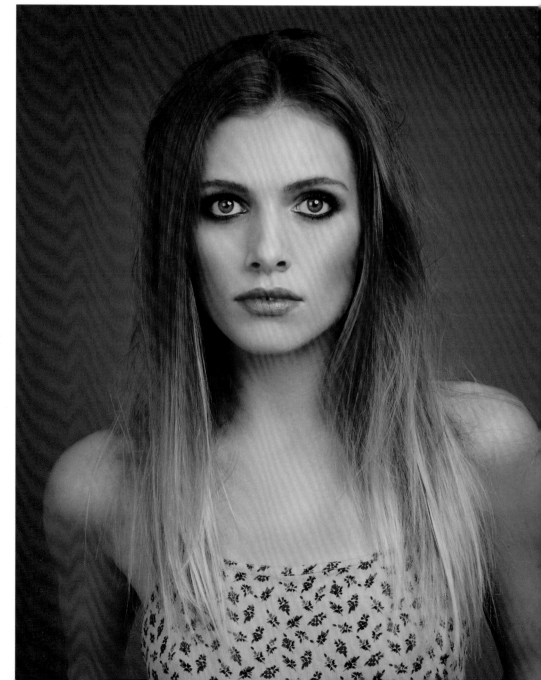

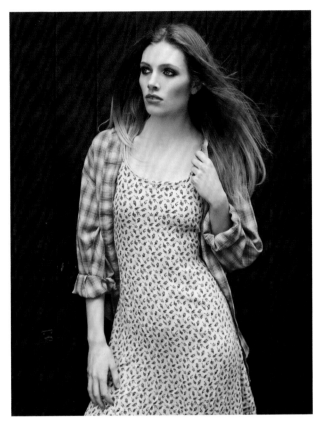

Make-up variation

Apply foundation, concealer and powder, as described on page 19.

Apply black kohl pencil all around the eyes and smudge with a cotton bud. Apply black kohl to the waterline and add black mascara. To keep this eye make-up longer, add black matte eyeshadow over the pencil around the eyes.

Shade the cheeks slightly darker, and use a raisin/plum-coloured stain on the lips.

Hair variation

A little texturizing spray was applied to tousle the hair.

Page numbers in *italics* are illustrations

1910s
  colours 16
  cosmetics *14*
  Gibson Girl 18–25
  make-up & hair 13
1920s
  colours 16
  cosmetics *15*
  look 1: 18–25
  look 2: 26–33
  look 3: 34–9
  look 4: 40–3
  make-up & hair 13, 69
1930s
  colours 50
  cosmetics *48–9*
  look 1: 52–7
  look 2: 58–61
  look 3: 62–5
  make-up & hair 47
1940s
  colours 72
  cosmetics *70–1*
  look 1: 74–7
  look 2: 78–81
  look 3: 82–5
  look 4: 86–7
  look 5: 88–9
  look 6: 90–3
  look 7: 94–7
  look 8: 98–101
  look 9: 102–5
  look 10: 106–9
  look 11: 110–13
  look 12: 114–17
  look 13: 118–23
  look 14: 124–7
1950s
  colours 134
  cosmetics *132–3*
  look 1: 136–9
  look 2: 140–3
  look 3: 144–5
  look 4: 146–51
  look 5: 152–7
  look 6: 158–61
  make-up & hair 131
1960s
  colours 168
  cosmetics *166–7*
  look 1: 170–7
  look 2: 178–81
  look 3: 182–7
  look 4: 188–91
  look 5: 192–5
  look 6: 196–201
  make-up & hair 165
1970s
  colours 208
  cosmetics *206–7*
  look 1: 210–15
  look 2: 216–19
  look 3: 220–5
  make-up & hair 205
1980s
  colours 232
  cosmetics *230–1*
  look 1: 234–9
  look 2: 240–3
  make-up & hair 229
1990s
  colours 232
  cosmetics *230–1*
  look 1: 244–7
  look 2: 248–9
  make-up & hair 229

A

advertisements 9
afros 165, 205, 220–5
Andress, Ursula *178*
Aniston, Jennifer 229
Arden, Elizabeth 13
Art Deco, influence on packaging *15*, *49*

B

Baby Doll lipstick *167*
'baby doll' look *192*
Bacall, Lauren *69*, 73
Bailey, David 196
Baker, Josephine 13
Ball, Lucille 73, 90
Bankhead, Tallulah *58*
Bara, Theda 16, 17, 26
Bardot, Brigitte *192*
Barrymore, Drew *248*
Biba
  Biba eyeshadow *207*
  Biba lipsticks 209
  Biba loose powder *207*
  Biba paintbox *207*
  Biba shampoo *206*
The Biba look 165, 216
Blend-Rite hairgrips *133*
blusher. *see also* rouge
  1920s 16, 20
  1930s 50
  1940s 72, 89
  1950s 134
  1960s 168, 184
  1970s 208
  1980s 232
  1990s 232

application 20, 184
  lipstick used as 103
  Madeleine Mono blusher *231*
the bob 13, *15*, 34–9, 165
  technique 37
Bourjois Endearing *132*
Bow, Clara *12*, 13, 34
Boyd, Pattie *192*
'boyish bob' *15*
Brooks, Louise 13, 17, *34*, 35
Brown, Bobbi 232
Buch + Deichmann clips *230*

C

The Castle bob 34–9
Castle, Irene 34
cinema, influence of 69, 70, 72, 131, 165, 205
clippers: French shingling clippers *15*
clips. *see* hair slides
Coddington, Grace 165
colours
  1920s 16
  1930s 50–1
  1940s 72
  1950s 134
  1960s 168
  1970s 208
  1980s 232
  1990s 232
compacts
  BOAC powder compact *132*
  combination compact *48*
  Geminesse powder, compact and cake liner *206*
  mirrored lip compact *133*
  wartime influence on *70*, *71*
concealer
  1920s 19, 35
  application 19
conditioner: Yardley hair conditioner *166*
contouring 168, 184
cosmetics
  1910s 13, *14*
  1920s 13, *15*
  1930s 47, *48–9*
  1940s 69, *70–1*
  1950s 131, *132–3*
  1960s 165, *166–7*
  1970s 205, *206–7*
  1980s 229, *230–1*
  1990s 229, *231*
  regulation introduced 50
  unregulated ingredients 13, 16, 47
cosmetics industry 13, 47, 69, 131, 166, 205, 206, 229
Coty airspun powder *48*
Crawford, Joan 73
Cupid's bow lips 17, 28, 236
curlers *70*, *106*. *see also* setting hair
curling 77, 91, 106, 141, 155, 237

'natural' curls 217
'cut crease' eye make-up 171, 178, 180, 189

D

Day, Doris *140*
Diana, Princess 229, 232
Dietrich, Marlene 47, 51
doe-eyed look 131, 134, 141
Donald's Velvette *14*
Dors, Diana 131
Dovima 131
Driscoll, Julie 165

E

The Egyptian look 40–3, 165
Ekland, Britt *182*
Elizabeth Arden 13
  Elizabeth Arden lashes *166*
eyebrows
  1920s 17, 27
  1930s 51, 53
  1940s 73
  1950s 135
  1960s 169
  1970s 209
  1980s 233
  1990s 233
  angled 73, 135
  arched 51, 53, 73, 75, 153
  blocking out 27, 169
  natural 211, 233
  shaping 27, 35
  straight 35
  thickening 235
  thin 209
eyelashes. *see also* mascara
  Elizabeth Arden lashes *166*
  eyelash beading *14*
  false 76, 100, 109, 153, 165, 168, 173, 193, 211
  Helena Rubinstein false lashes *133*
  painted on 168, 178
eyeliner
  1940s 72
  1950s 141
  1960s 168
  application 76, 141, 153, 171, 183
  flicked 72, 134, 165, 171
eyeshadow
  1920s 16, 19, 28
  1930s 50, 53
  1940s 72
  1950s 134
  1960s *167*, 168
  1970s 208
  1980s 232
  1990s 232
  application 19, 28, 75, 173, 221

Biba eyeshadow *207*
Marks & Spencer make-up *230*
Pond's eyeshadows *167*
Revlon Ultima eyeshadow *231*

F

face powder. *see* compacts; powder
false lashes. *see* eyelashes
Farrow, Mia *165*
Fashion Fair *208*
Fawcett, Farrah *204, 205, 210*
femme fatale look *16*
finger waves: technique *55*
First World War, influence of *13*
Flappers *13*
flicked up hair *185, 200*
Flori Roberts *208*
Fonssagrives, Lisa *131*
Fontaine, Joan *146*
foundation
    1920s *19, 20, 35*
    application *19*
    Mary Quant foundation *206*
    Max Factor Creme Puff *132, 133*
    Max Factor Pan-Cake *47, 70, 72*
    Max Factor Pan-Stick *71, 182*
    for women of colour *208*
freckles, drawn on *199*
French pleat *147, 189*
French shingling clippers *15*
fringes *110, 111, 114, 158*

G

Garbo, Greta *47*
Gardner, Ava *69, 106*
Garland, Judy *82*
Gibson, Charles Dana *18*
Gibson Girl style *18–25*
Gladys Cooper face powder *15*
Grable, Betty *69, 88, 90*
Grace, Princess of Monaco. *see* Kelly, Grace
Grateau, Marcel *15*
Gray, Coleen *86*
The Great Depression *47, 69*
grunge look *229, 232, 248–9*

H

hair accessories *22, 64, 92, 149, 193, 229*
hair slides *70, 230*
hair styles. *see also* individual styles e.g. bob
    1910s *13*
    1920s *13*
    1930s *47*
    1940s *69*
    1950s *131*
    1960s *165*

    1970s *205*
    1980s *229*
    1990s *229*
hairgrips: Blend-Rite hairgrips *133*
hairpieces *165, 174, 193*
Hall, Jerry *205*
Hampden rouge *49*
Harlow, Jean *47*
hats, influence of *13, 47, 58, 69, 131, 140, 148*
Hayworth, Rita *69, 78, 94, 106*
Helena Rubinstein *13*
    waterproof mascara *47*
Hepburn, Audrey *131, 135, 158*
hippy-influenced styles *165, 169*
Hollywood glamour style *52–7*
Hunt, Marsha *220*
Hunter's Bow lips *73*
Hurrell, George *69*
Hutton, Lauren *231*

I

Iman *230*
'Italian Boy' cut *131*

J

Jones, Grace *205*

K

Kelly, Grace *130, 136, 170*
Kiss Me lipsticks *132*
Kwan, Nancy *165*

L

Lake, Veronica *69, 94*
Lamour, Dorothy *62, 118*
Lauper, Cyndi *234*
Le Bon, Yasmin *229*
lip rouge *13*
lip stencils *28*
lipgloss *16*
lips
    1920s *17*
    1930s *51*
    1940s *73, 122*
    1950s *135, 154*
    1960s *169*
    1970s *209*
    1980s *233*
    1990s *233*
    Cupid's bow *17, 28, 236*
    Hunter's Bow *73*
    rosebud shape *51*
    rounded *73, 122*
lipsticks
    1920s *16, 20*
    1930s *54*

1940s 72, 85
1950s 134
1960s 167, 168
1970s 208
1980s 232
1990s 232
application 20, 54, 76, 222
  Baby Doll lipstick 167
  Kiss Me lipsticks 132
  Madeleine Mono lip colour 231
  Mary Quant Special Recipe lipstick 207
Lockwood, Margaret 133
Lollobrigida, Gina 131, 144
Lombard, Carole 47
London It Girl 196
Loren, Sophia 144, 188
Loy, Myrna 52

M

MAC Cosmetics 229
Madeleine Mono blusher 231
Madeleine Mono lip colour 231
Madonna 229
magazines, influence of 47, 50
make-up. see cosmetics; individual types e.g. mascara
Mansfield, Jayne 131
Marcel wave irons 15
Marcel waves 29–32, 33, 41
Margaret, Princess 124
Marks & Spencer make-up 230
Mary Quant
  Mary Quant foundation 206
  Mary Quant make-up 167
  Mary Quant Special Recipe lipstick 207
mascara
  1910s 14
  1930s 53
  1940s 75, 83, 114
  1980s 235
  coloured 235
  Maybelline cake mascara 49
  Ricil's cake mascara 49
  Rimmel mascara 71
  Rodier cake mascara 49
  waterproof 47
Max Factor 13, 14
  Creme Puff 132, 133
  Geminesse powder, compact and cake liner 206
  Geminesse range 208
  Lip Pomade 16
  Maxi range 205
  Pan-Cake foundation 47, 70, 72
  Pan-Stick 71, 182
Maybelline
  Maybelline cake mascara 49
  Maybelline mascara 14
Miranda, Carmen 114
models 131, 165, 196, 229

Monroe, Marilyn 131, 152
Moon, Sarah 205
Moss, Kate 229, 244
Murray, Mae 13
Musidora 16

N

natural look 165, 229, 244–7
natural products 206, 207
Nesbit, Evelyn 18

O

Ojos Negros powder 15

P

packaging
  1910s 14
  1920s 15
  1930s 48–9
  1940s 69, 70–1
  1950s 132–3
  1960s 166–7
  1970s 206–7
  1980s 230–1
  1990s 231
  Art Deco influence 15, 49, 207
  wartime influence 69, 70–1
padding out hairstyles 69, 120
pageboy hairstyle 137
Parker, Suzy 131
Patchett, Jean 131
peekaboo hairstyle 94–7
perfume: Charlie perfume 205
perming 229, 237, 238
pin curls 69, 97, 106
  technique 55
plaited hair styles 63
pompadours 21
Pond's
  Pond's eyeshadows 167
  Pond's make-set 166
ponytail 158–60
  setting hair 179, 193
pop music, influence of 131, 165, 205, 220, 229, 248
powder 48. see also compacts
  1910s 14
  1920s 14, 15, 35
  application 19, 35
  Biba loose powder 207
  BOAC powder compact 132
  Bourjois Endearing 132
  Coty airspun powder 48
  Gladys Cooper face powder 15
  Ojos Negros powder 15
  Tokalon loose powder 15
Prevost, Marie 26
punk, influence of 205, 229

Q

Quant, Mary 165, 166

R

Revlon
   Charlie make-up/perfume 205
   Revlon Face Gleamers 168
   Revlon Ultima eyeshadow *231*
Ricil's cake mascara *49*
Rimmel mascara *71*
Roberts, Julia *228, 234*
Rodier cake mascara *49*
Rogers, Ginger *46, 62*
rollers. see curling; setting hair
rolls 79, *88, 99*, 111
   The Victory Roll 118–19
The Ronettes 188
rosebud shape lips 51
Ross, Diana 205
rouge. see also blusher
   1910s 13
   1920s 16, 20
   1930s 50
   Hampden rouge *49*
Rubinstein, Helena 13
Russell, Rosalind *110*
Ryan, Meg 229

S

Sade *240*
Sassoon, Vidal 165
scarves as hair decoration 193
scrunch-drying hair 237
Second World War 69, 70, 87
setting hair 77, 91, 95, 99, 111, 155, 213, 237
   flicked up style 184
   ponytail 179, 193
   The Victory Roll 118–19
   waved pageboy 137
shampoo: Biba shampoo *206*
Sheppard, Lou 6, 9
Shields, Brooke 229, *234*
shingle haircut 15
Shrimpton, Jean *164, 166, 196*
slides. see hair slides
'smouldering' eyes 28, 40
The Spice Girls 229
Stefani, Gwen 229
supermodels 196, 229, 231, 244
switches 63, 240

T

Tangee
   Tangee lipstick 16
   Tangee make-up set *71*
tanned skin 15, 47, 209
Taylor, Elizabeth *98, 124, 131*, 165
teenage market 131, 158, 165
television, influence of 131, 205, 210, 229
Tierney, Gene 69, *74, 102*
Tokalon loose powder 15
Torres, Raquel *40*
transformations 13
turbans 216–19
Turlington, Christy *244*
Twiggy 165, 168, *216*

V

vamp look 26–32
Verushka 165
The Victory Roll 118–19

W

wartime influences 9, 13, 47, 69, 70, 103
wave clips *48*
waving
   finger waves 55
   Marcel waves 29–32, *33, 41*
   setting hair 77, 95, 99, 111, 137, 213
   waved pageboy 137
wefted hair 174
Welch, Raquel 192
Willcox, Toyah 234
Williams, Thomas Lyle *14*
Winehouse, Amy 188
women of colour
   1970s 220–5
   1980s 240–3
Women's Suffrage Movement 13

Y

Yardley hair conditioner *166*

Author's acknowledgements

I would like to thank the fantastic team who worked so hard on the book – Denisa, Madeleine, Cate, Dan.

Thank you to Elle, Grace, Rob, Nicky and family for always being enthusiastic about my projects!

My friend Wendy for all the support and encouragement. Thanks also to Carrie, Joe, Alex, Xabier, Zia, Daniel Crawford.

To our models Maddie, Shenise, Ellie, Georgie, Georgia, Lillie, Jasmine, Tiff, Elina, Emma, Rose, Hannah and Vanessa. Thanks also to to Wendy, Urte and Lauren.

Thanks to London Cosmetics Museum, Lulu Vintage Clothing, Past Caring, The Gallery Haircutters, 38 St Giles, The Assembly House in Norwich, Georgian Town House, Deco Days and Profile Models.

And of course thank you to Lou for sharing your amazing knowledge and skills.

Retouching: Denisa Ilie
Additional retouching: Annie Hawkes
Photography Assistants: Daniel Gregory and Andrew Parsons
Assistant: Rebecca Jennings

Models:

Elina: Early Years Look 3 (pp34–39) and Look 4 (pp40–43)

Ellie: 1940s Look 10 (pp106–8), 1950s Look 6 (pp158–61)

Emma: 1950s Look 5 (pp152–7)

Georgia: 1950s Look 1 (pp136–9), 1960s Look 3 (pp182–7) and Look 4 (pp188–91)

Georgie: p4, 1940s Look 6 (pp90–3), 1960s Look 6 (pp196–201)

Hannah: p7, 1940s Look 14 (pp124–27)

Jasmine: p8, Early Years Look 2 (pp26–33), 1930s Look 1 (pp52–7) and Look 2 (pp58–61), 1950s Look 2 (pp140–3) and Look 3 (pp144–5)

Lillie: Early Years Look 1 (pp18–25), 1940s Look 8 (pp98–101) and Look 9 (pp102–5), 1980s Look 1 (pp234–9)

Maddie: 1960s Look 1 (pp170–77), Look 2 (pp178–81) and Look 5 (pp192–5), 1990s Look 1 (pp244–7) and Look 2 (pp248–9)

Rose: 1970s Look 3 (pp220–5), 1980s Look 2 (pp240–3)

Shenise: Front cover, 1940s Look 1 (pp74–6), Look 2 (pp78–81), Look 3 (pp82–4), Look 4 (pp86–7), Look 5 (pp88–9), Look 7 (pp94–6), Look 11 (pp110–13), Look 12 (pp114–17) and Look 13 (pp118–23), 1950s Look 4 (pp146–51), 1970s Look 2 (pp216–19)

Tiffany: 1930s Look 3 (pp62–65)

Vanessa: 1970s Look 1 (pp210–15)

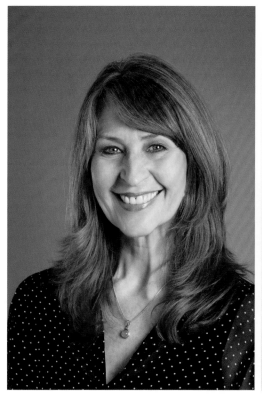

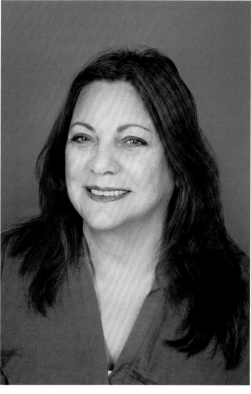

Louise Young

Louise has worked as a professional makeup artist in film, television and fashion for over 35 years and has written courses and qualifications in make-up that are taught throughout the UK. Louise works on leading film and TV productions and has made up some of the best-known faces in the entertainment industry. She also has her own range of brushes and cosmetics.

Loulia Sheppard

Lou is one of the film industry's leading hairstylists. Working on numerous award-winning productions, she has been personal hairstylist to some of the world's biggest stars, including Scarlett Johansson and Keira Knightly.